Inspirational Stories and Wisdom

Let's Talk About The C Word

How Cancer Gave More Than It Took

by
Shauna Marie MacDonald

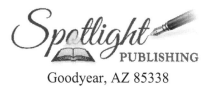

PUBLISHING
Goodyear, AZ 85338

MacDonald, Shauna Marie
Let's Talk About the C Word – How Cancer Gave More Than It Took – Inspirational Stories and Wisdom

ISBN: 978-1-7334077-3-1 Hardcover
ISBN: 978-1-7334077-2-4 Paperback
ISBN: 978-1-7334077-4-8 eBook

Cover Design: Adobe Images | Angie Anayla
Copyediting: Becky Norwood
Proofreading: Mark Norwood
Interior design: Anna Goldsworthy
Published by Spotlight Publishing™ www.SpotlightPublishing.Pro

Medical Disclaimer: Always consult your physician before beginning any auxiliary health and wellness program. This general information is not intended to diagnose any medical condition or to replace your healthcare professional. Consult with your healthcare professional to design an appropriate health and wellness prescription. If you experience any pain or difficulty with these practices, stop and consult your healthcare provider.

Inspirational Stories and Wisdom

Let's Talk About The C Word

How Cancer Gave More Than It Took

by
Shauna Marie MacDonald

Table of Contents

Acknowledgements

First and foremost, I want to thank my daughters Jaclyn St. Louis, Andrea Aesie, and Breanne Aesie. It is with your support and endless encouragement that this book lives today.

To Ron Aesie for giving me the inspiration through the lessons you shared with me in genuine integrity and truth.

To my darling friends who never gave up on me while I birthed this book. You listened to my chapters, continued believing in me and my vision, even when I'd disappear for weeks, failed to return your messages or canceled our plans together. Your love and support has been a constant source of amazement: Maddie Moss, Terry McGrath, Bonnie Earl, Myrna Brown, Janice Knight, Laurence Tessier, Henry VanAiken, Scott Brandon, Alex Kaganov, Lorna Corraini, Gyorgy Szabo, Christine Keillor, Vickie Hall, Colette Flemming, Janice Kulych, Karen Wallace-Fraser, Tanya Kelloway, Max Morin, Laurie Skreslet, Liz McKay, Charlie Vanderwilt, Betty MacDonald, and Deb Hagen.

To my editors and book designers who worked tirelessly to turn my vision into something exceptional: Julie Burton, Michael Wright, Becky Norwood, and team.

My publishers: Spotlight Publishing™ with Becky Norwood,

Natalie McQueen and their entire team of their creatives. You made this a delightful experience, even when I taxed your patience with delays. Not once did you complain or make me feel I was a burden. My deepest gratitude to you both. Your expertise and guidance were a constant source of comfort.

To all you lovelies I've interviewed for this book. It was a privilege to be in your presence. Your honest and open responses to my questions fed my passion for this book. You inspired me personally and now the world will know how truly amazing you are: Jen Gardiner, Jim Button, Barbra Marx Hubbard, Tim Ding, Charlie Scopoletti, and Luisa.

Inspiration for using the Dandelion on the book cover comes from a broader definition of the common and humble Dandelion which has a surprising amount of different meanings.

The Dandelion means:

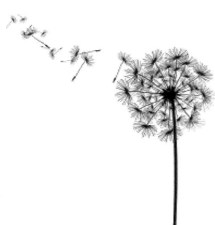

Healing from emotional pain and physical injury.

Intelligence, especially in an emotional and spiritual sense.

The warmth and power of the rising sun.

Surviving through all challenges and difficulties. Long-lasting happiness and youthful joy.

Getting your wishes fulfilled.

Since the Dandelion can thrive in difficult conditions, it is no wonder that people say the flower symbolizes the ability to rise above life's challenges.

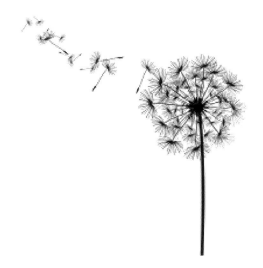

Introduction

Twirling in Italy

In January 2010, I had a burning desire to drop everything and go live in Florence, Italy. I'd been dreaming of Tuscany for as long as I could remember. As a teen, I was fascinated by the culture, ancient stone buildings, renaissance art, not to mention the pure romance of Italy's language and culture. When our three daughters were young, my ex-husband Ron and I, repeatedly discussed taking a year to live in the birthplace of da Vinci, Michelangelo, and Dante. As the years passed and the girls grew: excuses, circumstances, and roadblocks blurred our vision from our idealistic dream. But it was on this ordinary day, where the dream came bubbling to the surface, without overthinking it, I answered with a resounding YES.

I had no idea how, I just knew that if I kept walking in the direction of my dreams, the conditions and circumstances would miraculously present themselves. My fresh vision was of me waking up on my 49th birthday with a view of Tuscany outside my window. Sensible Shauna interjected with justifications of why I should not go. Fortunately, romantic Shauna prevailed.

The five weeks leading to my departure were a blur, but the details effortlessly fell into place:

- ✓ I found an apartment at an artist retreat in the hills of Tuscany.
- ✓ I temporarily closed my interior decorating business.
- ✓ Mere days before leaving, the perfect couple applied to rent my home filled with all my cherished possessions.

As a reminder that I was making an audacious commitment, an enthusiastic consortium of imaginary butterflies swirled within.

One of the benefits of embarking on an unexpected adventure is that you are afforded the luxury of witnessing the bounty of love and support from family and friends, no matter how impossibly tall you've built your castle in the sky. I was met with mostly positive reactions. I suspect behind closed doors, those closest to me wondered if I needed to be examined by a professional. But in truth, I rarely asked others for their opinion. This was something I was doing for me. The fiercely independent, tenacious, girl that lives just under my analytical surface, became focused and determined to turn this once-abandoned dream into reality.

The day arrived. As I settled into my seat next to the window, the flight cabin door closed with a resounding WHOMPH. In that moment, I could feel a shift from my life BEFORE, to the boundless potential of AFTER.

As I studied the view from my window, comfort and ease slipped silently from reach...adventure, mystery and the kaleidoscope of butterflies were buckled into the seat with me.

I inhaled one last breath of the familiar.

A cross between a smile and a smirk bloomed in the anxious corners of my lips...It was a SMIRKLE. Any lingering apprehension vanished as I sipped a glass of Chianti, or was it three?

In the weeks and months to come, as I navigated the animated, bewildering and interwoven texture of Italy, I came to associate the ever-present SMIRKLE, that would appear lovingly on my face. It was as a reminder to slow down, be curious, and observe the grace and guidance offered by every person, experience and happening.

My landlady, Federica was the first of many guides who drifted between mentor, caregiver, and friend. From the moment we met, Federica and I had a genuine bond. She owned the artist retreat where I lived for two months. It was January in Italy and in my first four weeks, I was the only occupant in her Italian haven, which was situated along the winding road of Via del Palmerino.

The week after my arrival I developed a determined flu. I was experiencing the exact symptoms of the highly infectious Swine Flu that was sweeping the globe that year. Federica offered to drive me to the doctor, but instead of a medical office, we arrived at the local pharmacy. I was curious but reasoned the doctor's office must be located behind the storefront.

What transpired next would prove to be the reason I'd come to Italy. With Federica's help translating, the pharmacist asked about all my symptoms, then respectfully plunged into a baffling inquiry. The first question Federica translated to me was:

Why did you come to Italy?

With a SMIRKLE on my face, I replied, "It has always been a dream to live in Italy."

I listened as Federica wove my words into Italian. The pharmacist seemed pleased with my answer and continued her inquiry:

Are you married?
"I've been divorced for six years."

Do you have children?
"I have three grown daughters."

Do you have a good relationship with them?
"Most of the time, yes!"

Have you explored Florence?
"A little, but then I got sick."

Do you have friends here?
"No"

Then came the final question, and it was a doozy:
Do you have a lover?

Seriously?? I looked at the ceiling for a hidden camera. I was sure I'd landed on some bizarre version of Italian Candid Camera. As if she'd asked a perfectly normal question, the pharmacist and

Twirling in Italy

Federica waited patiently for my response...

My exhausted and fuzzy brain yielded with weary surrender, "NO! I don't have a lover!! What exactly do any of these questions have to do with illness?"

What I really wanted to say was, "If I had a lover, he would be feeding me frozen gelato to combat my fever, and I certainly wouldn't be here answering these ridiculous questions".

The pharmacist disappeared behind a row of white metal shelves lined with amber bottles and meticulously arranged boxes. Distinctive notes from the theme of The Twilight Zone buzzed in my head. I had a thought: "is it possible to be aware when you're dreaming?" Absently, I lifted a fatigued hand to my head, bone-weary fingers brushed my forehead. The warmth confirmed a fever. There was no mistaking it, I was, in fact, awake, and standing in a pharmacy, in Italy...

"Where was the Doctor? I need a Doctor!!" I thought to myself.

The pharmacist returned with several prescriptions, complete with dosage and frequency. It was unlike any protocol I had ever come across. Keep in mind, this was all being translated to me, so I had time to process what she was saying. But it would be years before I'd fully understand the depth and insight of what she was actually dispensing:

- ✓ Take one zinc cough drop every three hours – savour it
- ✓ Rest and relax
- ✓ Research all the places you want to visit in Florence
- ✓ Sit on the stone bench in the garden with your bare feet in the grass

✓ Dance or twirl in the grass

My Smirkle vanished, replace by irritation.

The pharmacist then turned to Federica with a prescription for her to follow; she was to throw a party in my honour. Federica was to invite any neighbours and friends that she thought I might enjoy.

With a genuine smile, the pharmacist touched my hand, assuring me I'd be feeling better in a few days.

Federica and I walked out of the pharmacy. Sensing my uncertainty, she offered to take me to see a doctor. Between this last bewildering encounter, my persistent fever and deepening fatigue, I asked her to simply take me back to my room. In the following days, Federica lovingly cared for me, feeding me a steady diet of brown rice, homemade broth, and friendship. She explained who was invited to the party and why, shared her ideas for the menu, and set the dining room table for the festivities Saturday night.

For my part, I allowed my imagination as well as my body to dance, and on that first afternoon, I raised myself up to my feet and twirled. I must say it was a pathetic attempt. Hovering between embarrassment and skepticism, I had little to no belief that twirling in my bare feet would help my cough and fever. But, in the days to follow, I eventually found my footing and the confidence to fearlessly dance alone in the grass. Those afternoons twirling unconstrained in the garden became a delightful inner and outer adventure. In addition:
    ✓ I lowered my skepticism around the seemingly strange
       prescription.
    ✓ I savoured each Zinc cough drop.

- ✓ I rested and enjoyed the view of the green meadow out-side my window.
- ✓ I smiled often and to my surprise, I was actually healing.
- ✓ I sat on the stone bench every afternoon as the sweeping Tuscan sun set over the garden.
- ✓ I opened my heart and mind as my toes caressed the cool grass.

I merged my dreams and intentions for this trip onto an elegant sheet of embossed Italian stationary. It was titled:

Life in Italy

- ✓ A group of heart-centred international friends
- ✓ Cooking classes
- ✓ Italian lessons
- ✓ Daily smirks bubbling up from my very soul
- ✓ Bike rides along the Arno River
- ✓ Leisurely walks on stone-lined streets
- ✓ Guided trips to the museums of Florence
- ✓ Weekly visits to gaze upon Michelangelo's David.
- ✓ I wanted to figure out how it is when you have kindness, passion, and friendship in your life, healing follows.
- ✓ And why not throw in a handsome Italian to spice things up a little...

Saturday arrived, and with it one of my wishes was revealed. The guests were diverse, open-minded and became an instant community. Over time, they would come to share their individual brilliance, offering answers to all my questions on health, love, art, and adventure as I navigated my way through the Italian culture:

Gyorgyi – a philosopher and healer from Hungary

Peter – a dancer out of London

Monica – an art-historian and Italian linguist from Egypt

Donatella – a designer born in Florence, not to mention, Federica and her husband Stefano

My Italian adventure that appeared under twirling feet, would quickly become a tapestry of memories, weaving elegantly through the fabric that was my life.

Ten months later, I stood on the platform at the train station, where this family of friends bid me a teary farewell. My heart and eyes overflowed with emotions. It was then I understood why the pharmacist had me search out a community, examine my purpose, embrace the simple, connect to my surroundings, release any preconceived judgments and honour my beliefs. Through my Italian community, I inherited the wisdom of understanding that we are all connected in ways that are invisible to the eye, that healing originates in your core and moves outward. And with a little trust, you can grow, evolve and heal from the most unlikely of sources.

Returning to Canada, my life expanded in new directions, and with it, the gap widened between me and my Italian life. Memories of the Tuscan sun faded, and I didn't think about twirling, except on special occasions. One day without warning a reminder shot rang out.

Ron, the father of our three children, and my ex-husband was diagnosed with terminal cancer. My participation in his year of endings was negligible until the final eight weeks. It was then I realized that that our daughters, who were caring for him around the clock, were living on pizza and take-out. The basic need for healthy food was being grossly overlooked. I knew this was my opportunity to help. I made some calls to extended family and friends who were willing to drop off nourishing meals on a rotational basis. This also gave me an unanticipated opportunity to have quiet conversations with Ron in those final weeks. I was grateful he agreed to my perceived intrusion on his precious time with the girls. His generosity gave me an open window that afforded us closure on our history together.

On one such visit, we were having a straightforward conversation about our daughters, our 26-year marriage, and his wishes for the future of the family he was leaving behind, and he said something that would alter the course of my life and become the infrastructure upon which I based this book. He revealed to me that despite the hardship associated with his terminal illness, that for him, "Cancer Gave More Than It Took." He was grateful for the hours of laughter he'd had with the girls since his diagnosis. The vacations they had taken, their one-on-one conversations, and how sharing the amusing and difficult events of his life, without pretence, was curiously liberating.

Can you imagine, knowing you were arriving at the final chapter of your life, and opening-up with such dignity and acceptance? Ron passed away less than a week after that pivotal conversation.

In the months that followed, I returned to my beloved Florence and I couldn't stop wondering if there were others who had similarly experienced learning from cancer and what they believed had to shift in order to achieve this level of insight? More importantly, deciphering how others could achieve similar results. The foundations of *Let's Talk About The C Word: How Cancer Gave More Than It Took*, offers resources and uncomplicated methods to help uncover and identify what is essential for you to live phenomenally. Not only for cancer patients, but for their loved ones, friends, and caregivers too.

My experience in Italy taught me how to look for the gems behind adversity. How to twirl in order to see your life from all angles, not take anything for granted and to find gratitude and healing in unlikely places.

This book is dedicated to the memory of Ronald Michael Aesie and that of his three daughters, Jaclyn, Andrea, Breanne and five grandchildren who thrive with his humour, infectious laugh, and boundless optimism.

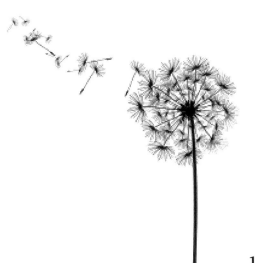

1.   I Choose Love

Jen Gardiner

Meeting Jen is like flipping on a switch in a darkened room. Her vivacious spirit infuses the space she occupies. Jen is warm, inviting, honest, witty – and you want her to be your best friend. Between an outrageous collection of hats, quirky clothing, hairstyles, a unique take on ANY situation, and her absolute belief in living in the moment, it's easy to fall in love with who she is, inside and out. It is my pleasure to introduce you to the effervescent Jen Gardiner.

Jen...

I knew I had cancer before my diagnosis, I just knew it. When the doctor told me the news, I had a moment where I held my breath, then I thought, 'Yeah, ok...this is the shits, but what do we do now?

I have stage 4 colorectal cancer. I was diagnosed on December 15, 2011. I'd been sick on and off with gut issues for the prior six months.

However, that wasn't anything out of the ordinary due to the fact I have ulcerative colitis. For twenty-seven years I was accustomed to colonoscopies, intestinal flare-ups, and medication. It took me some time to pay attention to the symptoms because of the underlying colitis. It became necessary to listen to my body when I landed in the hospital with a full bowel blockage.

A colonoscopy fourteen months prior showed no sign of cancer. The tumour itself just went KABOOM and blocked the large bowel. It burst through the walls of my insides, like paint loaded up on a brush that you flick on a wall, the cancer splattered everywhere. After three major surgeries, ten radiation treatments, and thirty rounds of chemo, cancer has jumped into my jaw, which is not typical of colorectal cancer. The treatments continue.

Cancer has many well-known side-effects. What I found most profound was how it teaches you what you need to learn. People find it hard to believe me when I say, "Cancer is a gift." It doesn't have to be cancer in your life, it can be any hardship: family drama, work-related stressors, a bankruptcy, a chronic health issue, or whatever gives you cause for pain, anxiety, and distress. I believe you are best served by incorporating adversity when it shows up, welcoming it, by turning it into a positive in your life. Now, don't go looking for difficulties, if you live long enough, lessons will find you...

I also emphasize that I wouldn't change the last two years for anything. I don't like the fact that my life will be OR is severely shortened; then again, I could be hit by a bus tomorrow. I recognize there's a blessing in the words; "Newsflash: you're gonna die and it could be real soon."

For me, a cancer diagnosis was like a cosmic BOOM; right here, right now the living clock starts. I do everything within my power to make my life joyous. Everything to make my friends, family and the people around me feel loved and experience life WITH ME, doing the most mundane or subtle things.

When you're given the gift of seeing your life flash before you as I have, you suddenly become aware of the pivotal points in your life. Bam, bam, bam, memories start dashing in front of your eyes; to me, it felt good because of all the fun I've had. I'm content with my choices. I'm not afraid to die, I'm not. I am afraid of leaving the people I love, and of not being able to touch them or be with them. I also believe that I'll have the capacity to be a part of their lives in a different way.

Most people today have been touched by cancer in some way. The growth potential lies in how you decide to digest it, how you make it part of your life. I can imagine some people are angry for a lifetime – that brand of poison I can do without. Allowing anger to rule my life is not how I want to live the with family and friends – *I CHOOSE LOVE*

There will be sadness when I'm gone. My husband and brother are going to wrestle with it. They are typical males; they feel helpless because they are unable to go in there with a hammer and nails and make this better. Eventually, they'll find their way; I'm sure of it. I firmly believe that there is an existence beyond this body. I know that we are pure energy; we go on and our spirit can't be destroyed. I'm secure in the belief that there is something else that can be done on the other side. I can carry on and help energetically from the mystical beyond.

For now, cancer has taught me lessons I believe are worthy of incorporating into life, with or without an illness. These lessons are for patients, families, caregivers...anyone who wants to live a life filled with love.

The FIRST LESSON I learned was to listen:

Listen to your body: Listen to what it needs by learning to be vigilant for the signs. Your body has a lot to tell you; you need to be insightful enough to listen. If you tune into your body, you have all you need to know. Firstly, your body informs your gut (also known as your microbiome) and if you can tune in and listen, your microbiome is an excellent source for wisdom. Become aware of that intuitive voice going on inside; listen to what it has to say, without freaking out over every little pang.

Don't ignore emotional clues, because when you don't trust your body/gut, that's when unhappiness flourishes and illness has an opportunity to grab hold. I've always been a believer in trusting your gut instincts - don't ignore them. There have been times when I've second-guessed myself and that's when I've messed up. Learn to listen to your intuition, in terms of your physical self, your emotional self, and believe we are born with everything we need. God, Buddha, Alla, Divine, Infinite, Goddess or whatever higher power you follow. It's your work to learn to listen to the clues, and they come to you through intuition, and for many of us it shows up as a gut feeling.

When you just know.

The SECOND LESSON, and by far the MOST challenging I've had to learn was:

Letting people help me. I'm fiercely independent; my mother brought me up that way.

My overachieving personality took it to the extreme. Friends or acquaintances ask, "Can I do this? Can I help you with that? Is there something I can take off your plate? May I take you to your appointment? Can I bring you dinner?" I'd say, "no-no, I'm fine, I'm fine." I'm very appreciative of and honoured by the fact that people are here to help. But at first, I felt like a burden and I took it as a personal slight to my abilities: "Do you think I can't do it? Do you think I'm so sick I can't take care of myself?" "Well, I'm Jen, and I'm not that sick"!! This attitude is highly destructive to your health, your relationships, and how you'll experience whatever illness or stress you are currently facing.

It's all about finding a balance between having a semblance of control and learning to release that control. What I've realized is: when my friends are allowed to help me, they experience joy. They want to reach out, they want to be a part of my life. I've learned how to receive. Receiving gracefully has been another revelation for me. As an added bonus, it makes my friends happy; I can see it on their faces and feel it from their hearts.

The THIRD LESSON is not new to me, I embraced it early on in life, and it has since emerged as a necessity post-diagnosis:

Live Life Fiercely. Every day is twenty-four hours of potential for something spectacular to happen. Pack in as much as your health allows. On the flipside of taking it all in is the lesson that, getting rest is rejuvenating and equally vital for good health. For a time, I wasn't doing enough recharging. What I've come to learn is that resting is a joy in and of itself. I do my best to never feel guilty, but if I need to lie down and whimper a bit, I do. Sometimes you need a pity party: embrace and feel that pity, and then let go of it when it's served its purpose.

The FOURTH LESSON I've had to learn – and it's not without complications – is:

Get it right with those you love. Your parents, your kids, your partner, your friends. Seriously, stop wasting time being angry. If you can't come to terms with it, move on. Stop letting that anger control you.

The FIFTH LESSON is to:

Cultivate a passion in your life. Remember...cancer does not define you. A wonderful way to do that is through service. Share your lessons, and you will inspire those around you.

The UpLife Project: motivates and inspires me, it gets me out of bed when I'm feeling low. My illness has shown me my life purpose. Before I got sick, I was involved in social media and had been working with the phrase, *"Jen Unplugged."* Aesthetically I like the feel of 'unplugged', it spoke to me:

- ✓ *Unplugged* from What Society Expects of You
- ✓ *Unplugged* from Fear
- ✓ *Unplugged* from Judgement
- ✓ *Unplugged* from Anger
- ✓ *Unplug* and Embrace Being Yourself

After the cancer diagnosis my passion, living *Unplugged,* moved into the forefront. It became my mantra: don't be afraid, don't shrink, there's love, support, beauty, faith, and spirituality all around. Become unplugged from everything that holds you back and come into your own.

That's essentially what *Unplugged* means to me now. It grew from being a feisty kid. My personality was formed by the time I was eight years old. I wasn't your average kid.

I grew up believing I was the secret lovechild of Liberace and Cher and that I had been born a fabulous gay man in another life.

The essence of *Jen Unplugged* appeared early on; I knew what I was going to do, who I was going to be. Peer-pressure and bullying slowed the progress of who I was. The real me flew under the radar, yet I carried on with who I was. I knew I had something to do in life. I was always a little bit on the outer edge of things. I liked to dress up, I liked to play, I liked to say outrageous things, but I was always very kind and cognizant of others' feelings. Essentially, I was a pleaser, always ensuring everyone was happy. I'd put myself on the bottom of the list; if I was happy, that was great, if not, "Oh well, I'll deal with my own happiness later." Unfortunately, that's not how it works. Once I came into my own, life flowed along. Then I met and married Sean: he is the love of my life.

With the cancer diagnosis, I realized there was absolutely no reason for me to hold back now. I decided to make every single day count; it will be the most spectacular two years anybody has ever seen. You're hoping it's more, of course. I made it my mission to incorporate value into every moment, a little bit of passion into every day I'm alive.

It was liberating for me to come into my own, and 'surprise, surprise', people responded positively to it. Their reactions were, "You've got Stage Four cancer, yet you're going out and doing all these energizing things, it's so inspirational." My response was always, "Thanks, however, this is just me. I'd most likely be doing all these outlandish things if I didn't have cancer, and with a two-year expiration date stamped on my life, living has become a priority."

It doesn't have to be all dolled up in extravagant clothing, or over the top experiences. It can be having a glorious day in your home reading, appreciating nature, visiting with friends or cuddling on the sofa with your love while holding hands and watching your favourite television show. I find joy in the simple moments of life! I only have to think of them and my heart pulses...pure bliss even in my memories of living life on my terms, with joy and gratitude.

I believe our greatest challenges bring about our greatest opportunities. I want to leave this place better that when I came in, by bringing awareness to the cutting-edge research and the dedicated work at the Tom Baker Cancer Centre here in Calgary. It's through their clinical trials lives are being saved or extended. I've set up a foundation: the *Jen Unplugged Experience Fund* in the hope that my passion will carry on long after I'm gone.

My purpose is to make people more aware, to bring education and funding for cancer research. Serving others is first and fore-most; it brings me exceeding joy to reach out, inspire and touch people, help them live happier lives. These are simple things that have a huge ripple effect outward. You drop the stone of joy in your life and watch the waves spread throughout your world. It not only touches the next person but every person they touch.

I Choose Love

A unique perk cancer offered me was the opportunity to figure out who I really am. To be at peace with her and be happy and joyful. It taught me to spiritually define my place in this world, to know that things are going to be okay when I'm gone, and more importantly to accept the love of my family and friends. Some relationships fell away because of cancer. That's ok too. I understand it makes people uncomfortable or challenges them in ways I can't see. It's not personal.

Of course, I'd never be upset with others who are simply honouring their journey, however, it's not healthy, physically or mentally, to be in contact with challenging relationships. That's true in any situation in life. I concentrate on the 99% of wonderful that's gone on with the beautiful people in my life.

My husband, Sean for instance. We had been dating for two years before my diagnosis. He was very supportive and very determined about getting me to pay attention to the signs my body was giving me. He's tenacious about my health because I'm stubborn; he knew I needed a loving push.

When I was recovering from my first major operation, he got down on bended knee and proposed to me. I gave him an out in the form of a question, "Are you sure? There's a lot of crap coming up with all of this. I don't know if I'm going to live or die. I could be bald, it's gonna be shit." I couldn't resist his answer: "I'm not finished with you yet. I love you. I want to take care of you, and you can't do this on your own."

Sean's been there holding my hand through everything. It's not easy on him. Cancer is brutal on the caregivers. It's difficult for me, yet I feel somehow, that I have more control. Scientifically, I don't, so I take charge of the things I can control. I choose love, faith, spirituality, happiness, and joy. These are the things I have jurisdiction over, and I believe these are a big part of healing.

Sean, my mother, brother, nephews, and friends, on the other hand, have to stand on the outside and just keep their fingers crossed. They can't do anything about it, and it makes them crazy. I said to Sean after a treatment, "I'm so glad it's me." His reply was, "What are you talking about? I wish it was me!" I said, "Yes, I know, but I'm so glad it's me because if it was you, I'd go mental; I'd lose my mind." He quietly turned to me and said, "That's how I'm feeling." To say I'm blessed having Sean in my life is a gross understatement.

Of course, I succumb to fear every now and again; everybody gets scared. I've learned that you have to acknowledge your fear and face it head-on. I understand ignoring it, delaying, or believing that 'if I don't think about it, it's not going to happen' is not healthy. My experience with fear is: don't procrastinate or push it aside. It's very rewarding to be able to conquer fear. Usually, it's never as bad as I think it's going to be. Fear of death is a big one for everyone. Acknowledge it with, "I'm scared, I'm pretty damn scared of death." Then ask yourself:
- ✓ What is fearful about this?
- ✓ Why am I fearful about it?
- ✓ How's it going to change who I am?

You can conquer your fears by changing a few things or by not giving it the strength or credibility that a lot of fear has. March right through it. Fear is only as great as the power you give it. I choose to use fear to my advantage, turn it into something constructive. Fear is a great motivator for me, and I use fear instead of fear using me.

I Choose Love

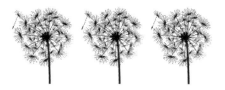

Jen Gardiner passed away on February 22, 2014, surrounded by love. Through her causes and vivacious spirit, Jen continues to be an inspiration.

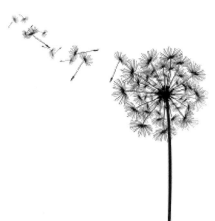

Happiness is the Cart ~ Love is the Horse

Jen chose to turn her fear into a positive attribute. She used fear, instead of it using and controlling her. How she did this was to concentrate on love, to make that her focus. It took courage and energy, plus some good old-fashioned work to find the good in life, but she made this her number one priority. Letting love in and embracing it each and every day.

One of the ways to flip our negative or fearful emotions to love is by going back in your mind to a time when you experienced the expansion of genuine LOVE, then expanding it further. Think of a time when you experienced:

✓ Romantic love
✓ Holding your child
✓ Discovering a life purpose
✓ Adopting a cherished pet

✓ A time you felt deep love in your life

When you find yourself engulfed in love, time expands, you have increased energy, require less sleep, your concentration is refocused, you experience a sense of joy, a surge in wellbeing and overall increased health. In this expanded state, two of the brain's neurotransmitters *(chemicals that communicate information throughout our brain and body, involved in the transmission of nerve impulses between nerve cells)* are activated.

The neurotransmitters associated with Love (Dopamine) and Happiness (Serotonin) are produced naturally in our bodies and bring with them an ability to assist in healing disease. When we are in a joyful love state our bodies work to heal us from within. Why? Because our mind & body resonate and heal in the energy of ease. Think of the word disease. Dis-(without) ease. Love brings us to a place of ease, and when your body is in a state of ease, you experience increased joy, health, and wellbeing. Of course, there are numerous elements involved with the healing process: trusted health providers, stress reduction, calm surroundings, outside support, acceptance, and belief in your healing.

Prioritizing what is important to you is a challenge in today's informed, yet ultimately disconnected world. The focus required to achieve a balance between healing protocols, relationships, career, home, family, and the desire to be connected to the outside world can be a staggering task. It's becoming increasingly more common for individuals to temporarily step back from the news, social media and public commitments. The constant barrage of incoming information has repercussions on one's ability to achieve balance and stability. Add fear, overwhelm, confusing medical terminology, not to mention the financial burden that often comes with illness, and you have a prescription for turmoil. These states of being are certainly not where healing resides.

With the diagnosis of an illness, you now have an excuse and a choice where you will focus your time and energy. You have the right to turn UP or turn OFF relationships and/or distractions, disconnect or reconnect on social media, use your cell phone to ask for help, or let it go to voicemail so you can be alone.

If people don't like it, that's not your concern. What they think of you is no longer your business. Your work, effort, and focus are on healing. Illness is the ultimate backstage pass to make decisions that work best for you. You've lost independence in one area of life: your health. I'm suggesting you implement guilt-free choices in areas of life that you do have some control over, your relationships. Take an inventory of who you spend time with – family, romantic partner, friends, as well as communities you are involved in. Decipher if they are nurturing your health or causing you additional suffering. Pull away from as many emotionally draining relationships as possible. It may be a temporary situation, just until your health improves.

An 80+ year scientific study has proven you can gain strength through close nurturing relationships. The relationships you have and the unexpected ones that grow as a result of illness have hidden potential.

The longest-running longitudinal study called, *The Grant-Glueck Harvard Study* found that the secret to leading a fulfilling life is directly tied to our relationships with others.

For over 80 years, the *Harvard Study* has tracked the physical and emotional well-being of two diametrically opposed populations: The Grant Study began in 1939, researchers followed 456 disadvantaged, non-delinquent inner-city youths who grew up in Boston neighbourhoods. The Glueck study followed 268 physically and mentally healthy men who were Harvard College sophomores from the classes of 1939–1944. One of them being U.S. president John F. Kennedy. *Women weren't in the original study because Harvard in the 1940s was all male.*

The Harvard Study, as the combined study is referred to today, is under its fourth director, Robert Waldinger. There are 59 of 724 subjects alive to date. The scope of the study has widened, it now includes the wives and children of the original participants. The significance of an analysis of this magnitude is that it has permitted the *study of time* on a diverse number of participants.

Due to the length of the research period, this has required multiple generations of researchers. Since before WWII, they have diligently analyzed blood samples, conducted brain scans (once available), pored over self-reported surveys, and engaged in one-on-one interactions with these men, their wives, and families, to compile the findings. No single interview, no single questionnaire is ever adequate to reveal the complete man, but the mosaic of interviews produced over many years has proven to be most revealing.

The conclusion, according to director Robert Waldinger, is that one key finding surpasses all the rest in terms of importance:

"The clearest message that comes from 80+ years of research: Good relationships keep us happier and healthier. Period!!"

It's not how big your bank account is, how successful your job, the size of your house, or how many likes you have on the photo you just posted on social media. Researchers who have pored through data, including vast quantities of medical records and hundreds of in-person interviews and questionnaires, found a strong correlation between participants who experienced flourishing lives and those who nurtured interactive relationships with family, friends, and community. Several studies found that people's level of satisfaction with their relationships at age 50 was a better predictor of physical health than cholesterol levels.

Robert Waldinger concludes in his TED Talk – *The Good Life*,

"When we gathered together everything we knew about them at age 50, it wasn't their middle-age cholesterol levels that predicted how they were going to grow old. The people who were the most satisfied in their relationships at age 50 were the healthiest at age 80. It was how satisfied they were in their relationships."

The most significant predictor of your happiness and overall fulfillment in life is LOVE.

Specifically, the *Harvard Study* demonstrates that having someone to rely on helps your nervous system relax, helps your brain stay healthier longer, and reduces both emotional as well as physical pain.

The data is also very clear that those who feel lonely are more likely to see their physical health decline earlier and die younger. Loneliness kills. It's as detrimental to your health as smoking, substance abuse or disease.

If you think running out and forcing friendships or remaining in a toxic marriage will work, Robert Waldinger reminds us,

"It's not just the number of friends you have or whether you're in a committed relationship. It's the quality of your close relationships that matters."

What this means is: Happiness and longevity are not based on whether you have a huge group of friends, go out every weekend, or if you're the most popular on social media. It's the quality of your relationships: how much vulnerability and depth exists within them, how safe you feel sharing with one another, the extent to which you can relax and the level of authenticity you share together.

According to George Vaillant, the Harvard psychiatrist who directed The Harvard Study from 1972 to 2004,

"There are two foundational elements to this: One is love. The other is finding a way of coping with life that does not push love away. For example: if you've found love and subsequently experience a trauma such as losing a job, the death of a parent or the loss of a child and you don't deal with that trauma, you could end up coping in a way that pushes that love away."

Let this be a reminder to prioritize not only your connection with others but your own capacity to handle emotions and stress. If you find yourself struggling, get help through a support group, enrol in a workshop, or see a grief counsellor. Take personal growth seriously in order to participate in relationships, they, in turn, keep you mentally and physically healthy.

The evidence is clear: you could acquire all the money you've ever dreamed of, have a successful career, be in top physical shape, but without loving relationships, the initial fulfillment these things bring quickly fades, and you'll be back striving for the next accomplishment. Even though relationships are messy, complicated and difficult and we are at times hurt and humbled by them, when we avoid and turn away from building healthy relationships, it's then that we lose.

Waldinger adds, "The surprising finding is that our relation- ships and how happy we are in our relationships have a powerful influence on our health. Taking care of your body is important but tending to your relationships is a form of self-care too."

The good life is built with good relationships.

A particular study of one of the participants in the *Harvard Study* was with 19-year-old Godfrey Minot Camille. He was a tall redheaded boy with a charming manner who planned to enter medicine or the ministry. In 1938, Camille was among the 268 Harvard College sophomores deemed by recruiters as likely to lead a "Successful Life".

Only gradually did the study's staff discover that the allegedly *normal* Godfrey was an intractable and unhappy hypochondriac. On the 10th anniversary of his joining the study, each man was given an A through E rating anticipating future personality stability. Godfrey's was assigned an E, the lowest possible rating.

But if Godfrey Camille was a disaster as a young man, by the time he was an old one he had become a star. His occupational success, measurable enjoyment of work, love, play, his health, the depth and breadth of his social support, the quality of his marriage and the relationships he shared with his children – all that and more combined to make him one of the most successful of the surviving men of the study. What made the difference? How did this sorry lad develop such an abundant capacity for flourishing?

These are the kinds of questions that can only be answered by a study that follows participants over the course of a lifetime. Through reviews of Godfrey and his Harvard peers', medical records, coupled with periodic interviews and questionnaires exploring their careers, relationships, and mental well-being, the study's goal was to identify key factors to a happy and healthy life.

This was certainly the case with Godfrey, whose life illuminates two of the most important lessons from the Study:

One is that happiness is love.
The other is that people really can change.

As we see in the example of Godfrey Camille's life, people really do have the capacity to grow.

From a bleak childhood: Godfreys' parents were upper class, but they were also socially isolated and pathologically suspicious. A child psychiatrist who reviewed Godfrey's record 30 years later, thought his childhood one of the bleakest in the Study.

Unloved, and not yet grown into a sense of autonomy, as a student Godfrey adopted the unconscious survival strategy of frequent reports to the college infirmary. No evidence of tangible illness was found at the majority of his visits and in his junior year, a usually sympathetic college physician dismissed him with the disgusted comment, "This boy is turning into a regular psychoneurotic." Godfrey's constant complaining was an immature coping style. He didn't connect with other people and it kept them from connecting with him; they didn't see his real under-lying suffering and just got angry at his apparent manipulations.

After graduation from medical school, the newly minted Dr. Godfrey Camille attempted suicide. The Study consensus at the time of his 10-year personality assessment, at the tender age of 29, was that he was "not fitted for the practice of medicine," and unloved as he was, he found taking care of other people's needs overwhelming. But several sessions with a psychiatrist gave him a different view of himself. Godfrey wrote to the Study, "My hypochondriasis has been mainly dissipated. It was an apology, a self-inflicted punishment for aggressive impulses."

Then, at age 35, he had a life-changing experience. He was hospitalized for 14 months in a veterans' hospital with pulmonary tuberculosis. Ten years later he recalled his first thought on being admitted: "It's neat; I can go to bed for a year, do what I want and get away with it."

Godfrey confessed, "I was glad to be sick," His illness, a real one, finally ended up giving him the emotional security that his childhood - along with his hypochondriacal symptoms and subsequent careful neutrality – never had. Dr. Godfrey Camille felt his time in the hospital almost like a religious rebirth. "Someone with a capital 'S' cared about me," he wrote. "Nothing has been so tough since that year in the sack."

Released from the hospital, Dr. Camille became an independent physician, married and grew into a responsible father and clinic leader. His coping style changed as the decades passed. His transitional reliance on displacement *(the unconscious avoidance of emotional intensity)* was replaced by the still more empathetic involuntary coping mechanisms of altruism and generativity *(a wish to nurture others' development)*. He was now functioning as a giving adult. Whereas at 30 he had hated his dependent patients, by 40 his adolescent fantasy of caring for others had become a reality. In vivid contrast to his post-graduation panic, he now reported that what he liked most about medicine was that, "I had problems and went to others, and now I enjoy people coming to me."

When Dr. Camille was almost 70, he was asked by George Vaillant, then director of the *Harvard Study*, what he had learned from his children. "You know what I learned from my children?" he blurted out, tears in his eyes. "I learned love!"

Many years later, having seized a serendipitous opportunity to interview Dr. Camille's daughter, Vaillant recounted that he believed him, "I have interviewed many *Harvard Study* children, her interview stood out because of her love for her father. It remains the most stunning that I have encountered among them."

At age 75, Godfrey, while being interviewed, took the opportunity to describe in greater detail how love had healed him.

"Before there were dysfunctional families, I came from one. My professional life hasn't been disappointing – far from it – but the truly gratifying unfolding has been into the person I've slowly become, comfortable, joyful, connected, and effective. Since it wasn't widely available then, I hadn't read that children's classic, The Velveteen Rabbit, which tells how connectedness is something we must let happen to us, and then we become solid and whole. As that tale recounts tenderly, only love can make us real. Denied this in boyhood for reasons I now understand, it took me years to tap substitute sources. What seems marvellous, is how many there are (in life) and how restorative they prove to be. What durable and pliable creatures we are, and what a storehouse of goodwill lurks in the social fabric...I never dreamed my later years would be so stimulating and rewarding."

That convalescent year, in hospital, transformative though it was, was not the end of Dr. Camille's story. Once he grasped what had happened, he seized the ball and ran with it, straight into a developmental explosion that went on for 30 years. A professional awakening and a spiritual one; a wife and two children of his own; two psychoanalysis, a return to the church of his early years – all these allowed him to build for himself the loving surround that he had so missed as a child and to give to others out of its riches.

At 82, Dr. Godfrey Minot Camille had a fatal heart attack while mountain climbing in his beloved Alps. His church was packed for the memorial service. "There was a deep and holy authenticity about the man," said the Bishop in his eulogy. His son summoned up his life, "He lived a very simple life, but it was very rich in relationships." Yet prior to age 30, Camille's life had been essentially barren of relationship. Folks change, but they stay the same, too. Camille had spent his years before the hospital looking for love, it just took him a while to learn how to do it well.

Lessons Learned on How to Flourish by *Harvard Study* director, George Vaillant: In 2009, Vaillant delved into the Harvard Study data to establish results he titled:

Decathlon of Flourishing
Citing a set of ten accomplishments that covered many different facets of success;

- ✓ Two of the items in the Decathlon of Flourishing had to do with Economic Success
- ✓ Four had to do with Mental and Physical Health
- ✓ Four with Social Supports and Relationships.

He then set out to see how these accomplishments correlated or didn't, with the three gifts of nature and nurture;

- ✓ Physical Constitution

- ✓ Social and Economic Advantage
- ✓ A Loving Childhood

The results were as clear-cut as they were startling.

They found that measures of family socioeconomic status had no significant correlation at all with later success in any of these areas. Alcoholism and depression in family histories proved irrelevant to flourishing at age 80, as did longevity. What was remarkable was that the sociability and extraversion that were so highly valued in the initial process of selecting the men did not correlate with later flourishing either.

In contrast with the weak and scattershot correlations among the biological and socioeconomic variables, a loving childhood – and other factors like empathic capacity and warm relationships as a young adult – predicted later success in all ten categories of the Decathlon of Flourishing. What's more, success in relationships was highly correlated with both Economic Success and Strong Mental and Physical Health, the other two broad areas of the Decathlon.

In short, *it was a history of warm intimate relationships – and the ability to foster them in maturity – that predicted flourishing in all aspects in the lives of the men studied.*

For instance, it was found that there was no significant difference between the maximum earned incomes of the men with IQs of 110–115 and the incomes of the men with IQs of 150- plus. On the other hand:

Men with warm mothers took home $87,000 more than those men whose mothers were uncaring.

Men who had good sibling relationships when young were making an average of $51,000 more a year than the men who had poor relationships with their siblings.

The 58 men with the best scores for warm relationships made an average of $243,000 a year; in contrast, the 31 men with the worst scores for relationships earned an average maximum salary of $102,000 a year.

When it comes to late-life success – even when success is measured strictly in financial terms – the finds that Nurture outperforms Nature. And by far the most important influence on a flourishing life is LOVE. Not early love exclusively, and not necessarily romantic love. But love early in life facilitates not only love later on, but also the other trappings of success, such as high income and prestige. It also encourages the development of coping styles that facilitate intimacy, as opposed to the ones that discourage it. The majority of the men who flourished found love before 30 and the data suggests that was why they flourished.

We can't choose our childhoods, but the story of Dr. Godfrey Camille reveals that a bleak childhood does not doom us. If you follow lives long enough, people adapt and they change, so do the factors that affect healthy adjustment. Our journeys through this world are filled with discontinuities.

Nobody in the *Harvard Study* was doomed at the outset, but nobody had it made either. Inheriting the genes for alcoholism can turn the most otherwise blessed golden boy into a skid row bum. Conversely, an encounter with a very dangerous disease liberated the pitiful young Dr. Camille from a life of loneliness and dependency. Who could have foreseen, when he was 29, and the

Harvard Study staff ranked him in the bottom 3% of the cohort in personality stability, that he would die a happy, giving and beloved man?

Only those who understand that **happiness is only the cart ~ love is the horse** and perhaps those who recognize that our so-called defence mechanisms, our involuntary ways of coping with life, are very important indeed. Before age 30, Dr. Camille depended on narcissistic hypochondriasis to cope with his life and his feelings; after 50 he used empathic altruism and a pragmatic stoicism about taking what comes.

The two pillars of happiness revealed by the 80+ year Harvard Study – and exemplified by Dr. Godfrey Minot Camille – are:

Pillar 1 – Focus on love and healthy love-based relationships.
Pillar 2 – Focus on a mature coping style that does not push love away.

Above all, the *Harvard Study* reveals how men like Dr. Camille adapted themselves to life and adapted their lives to themselves – a process of maturation that unfolds over time. The *Harvard Study* is an instrument that permitted the study of time, much as the telescope uncovered the mysteries of the galaxies and the microscope enabled the study of microbes.

For researchers, prolonged follow-up can be a rock upon which fine theories founder, but it also can be a means of discovering robust and enduring truth. At the outset of the Study in 1939, it was thought that men with masculine body types – broad shoulders and a slender waist – would succeed the most in life.

That turned out to be one of many theories demolished by the *Harvard Study* as it followed the lives of these men. To benefit from the lessons both of the *Harvard Study* and of Life requires persistence and humility. Without it, maturation makes liars of us all.

Links & Resources:
TedTalk on The Harvard Study –
https://www.youtube.com/watch?v=8KkKuTCFvzI

Harvard Study-Harvard Gazette:
http://news.harvard.edu/gazette/story/2017/04/over-nearly-80-years-harvard-study-has-been-showing-how-to-live-a-healthy-and-happy-life/

Article by George E. Vaillant, M.D
http://greatergood.berkeley.edu/article/item/what_are_secrets_to_happy_life/success

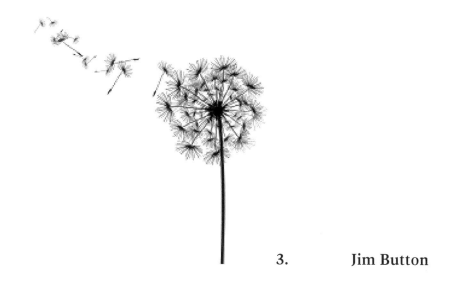

3.   Jim Button

Bubbles & Bathtubs

The week after celebrating finishing the manuscript for, "Let's Talk About The C Word," I stumbled upon a YouTube video called "Tub Talks," hosted by funnyman and Calgary local celebrity, Dave Kelly.

Picture this: a quirky interview that takes place between Dave Kelly and Jim Button, two men, submerged to the chest in a bubble bath. Now, keep in mind, it's a tub built for one, with a candle burning in the corner, a jumble of feet, elbows, knees, and legs, as they casually discuss topics such as: family, friends, marriage, cancer, the meaning of life, and how quickly bubbles disappear. I was struck by the unexpected brilliance of their location, while exploring issues conventional society dances around. It's refreshing how humour helps you relax and lean in toward a complex subject matter such a death, life and the value of a perfect ice-cream cone.

When I stumbled on the video, I was canning pasta sauce an was elbow deep in garlic, olive oil, and ripe tomatoes. A barrage of questions hit me at once:

- ✓ How did I miss this brilliant bathtub banter?
- ✓ Who is Jim Button?
- ✓ Should I add another chapter to my book?
- ✓ How could I not?

One week after watching this man have a bath surrounded with bubbles and his best friend, I met Jim Button. He breezed into the coffee shop for our interview. It was an overcast morning in November. Meeting Jim is like inhaling sunshine. He exudes natural joy that stems from core beliefs: happiness, integrity and community service. He radiates a natural charm despite his condition of stage 4 renal cell carcinoma – kidney cancer.

It is with delight and unyielding gratitude I share Jim Button's story.

Jim Button...

Cancer introduced itself while rafting on Father's Day. I wasn't feeling myself and was in a lot of pain. A few days later, I went to the doctor, who believed it was appendicitis. The standard tests were ordered, but instead of just the appendix being ruptured, they found a baseball-size tumour on my kidney.

Diagnosis: Renal cell carcinoma. I had my appendix removed and the following week, a kidney. I went home to recover. Not very much changed for me, and unless it came up, the majority of people didn't even know about the cancer. Life returned to normal.

It was at my third follow up CT scan when I knew I was in trouble. My wife and I went in for the results. The intern refused to look me in the eye, and the doctor motioned for me to sit down. In that moment, and in the hours to come, life shifted.

The interesting part for me is that I've always managed well when life doesn't obey our carefully constructed blueprint. My coping mechanism has always been to help others come to grips with what's going on through lighthearted humour. I have the ability to make others feel comfortable. My wife cried, the intern continued to stare at the floor, and I cracked jokes.

The cancer had spread to my lungs. Prognosis, one year to live.

My wife and I went home to absorb the news, even as positive as I am, the diagnosis rocked my world. I went through many emotions that afternoon. Then in a flash, reality as I knew it cracked wide open. It was a series of separate, yet interconnected situations that presented themselves to me, and I could listen or ignore the synchronicity of those two events.

I received a text from a good friend Avnish Mehta, a wise, aligned and spiritual human who openly shares his love of meditation and mindful living. Now normally, with everything going on, the average person wouldn't look at their phone, but something told me to read it. His text crystallized my belief in the mysterious connection that often exists between friends. He explained that during a meditation, he saw shadows around my lungs and thought I should have it looked at by my oncologist.

I was dumbfounded. Imagine the unlikelihood of the science-based medical community and the unexplained spiritual world coming to the same conclusion, individually within a few hours. On the medical side, I had the best scientific technology and doctors in the world working with me at the Tom Baker Cancer Centre here in Calgary. They had just diagnosed me with terminal lung cancer and within a few hours my friend from the spiritual/metaphysical world, with no prior knowledge of my oncologist appointment, shared with me that he saw an image of my lungs shrouded in shadows.

With the significance of those two events colliding, my health journey became an integrative co-creation. It was a distinct reminder that I didn't have to choose one over the other. My wife Tracey and I immersed ourselves in meditation, mindfulness and any alternative, woo-woo practices that felt right for us. We fully integrated science and spirituality, through the ever-shifting health reality that is cancer.

I chose complete transparency with anyone who cared to listen. I focused on what was right for me and chose not to get thrown off by the opinions of others. It is an evolving journey. The decisions pertaining to my health involve my wife Tracey, my children, and my health team, consisting of doctors, alternative health practitioners and those I trust with my life. I honour what I believe is in my best interest physically, emotionally and spiritually. Tracey's calming presence and unwavering support keeps me grounded, focused and on the straight and narrow. It's not easy for her, because my creative mind likes to wander and take detours. I don't always put myself, or my health first, so it's her mission to keep me on track.

Because of the treatments I was receiving, the most comfortable place for me was in the bath. Dave and I decided to do the interview in the tub because I wanted to change the dialogue around cancer and to do that, I had to get peoples' attention in a creative way. Talking about cancer is easy for me, I want others to discover that by speaking genuinely and with a degree of lightness, much of the fear and awkwardness falls away. When you've been diagnosed with an illness, let alone a fatal one, people talk about you behind your back. I'm here to tell you...no one likes that! I made the choice to get it out in the open. If it's not right for you to share your story, that's ok. There are no judgments here. However, I think you might enjoy what Dave and I have to say, and at least you'll have a chuckle watching a couple of naked guys make fools of themselves.

I also write a blog called GatherWithJim.com. It chronicles my journey, thoughts, and experiences. I write for patients, family, and friends unraveling the mystery, by tackling the fear through open and honest dialogue. In turn, it allows those who care about me, to know where I'm at in my healing, because a considerable amount of people won't or can't talk about cancer. I've found that for them, in reading about my experience, they have a better day.

Often, I'll feel like writing, but I have no idea what to write about. Once the words start flowing, I discover what needs to be said. I enjoy talking to others who are experiencing cancer. The connection is instant. I've made new friends as a result of my open dialogue and willingness to share. I have a new level of understanding: I want to live a life of purpose, a life of sharing and a life of meaning.

Years ago, I worked in advertising, I enjoyed the creativity of it and now that I own a business and participate in multiple community organizations, I need to be innovative in order to create a vision for the future for myself and my employees. I can't follow my vision when I'm slumped over feeling sorry for myself and wishing things had been different. Writing helps me stay focused, creative, and productive, especially during treatments and recovery. When life gets altogether too serious, I find the written word has the capacity to tap directly on my funny bone. Don't get me wrong, I'm fully aware of the consequences of cancer. My family and I are living it. I simply choose to be on the side of laughter, positivity, and possibility.

My motto is, *make each day matter.* I've always been a positive guy and an open book about most things. It's not difficult for me to share experiences with others and cancer is no different. I enjoy the connections I make. It's truly rewarding, and I find that when you are open and honest, the return is always greater than your output. I grew up in a household where we laughed a lot. My parents were equally pragmatic and wise about life. My mother was such a funny woman. She laughed about things most people considered serious. She was a nurse, so she had a healthy balanced attitude around illness.

One of the last conversations I had with my mother at the end of her own journey with cancer, was when I was lying beside her. I asked what the Top Three things she'd learned were. Even in her frail state, she laughed out loud. When I asked why she was laughing, she said she knew the question was coming and she also knew that out of her four sons, I'd be the one to ask: *These are my wise mother's Top Three Things to Remember in Life:*

"Be Nice ~ Life is Easy ~ Laugh a Lot"

You see, even death isn't the end if you get to that point where you understand that the *energy component* of who we are lives on. I don't happen to believe in a lot of goings-on after death, but I do understand that energy lingers long after we're gone. With this awareness, I'm making sure the momentum I've created lives on.

44

I'm a believer in legacy. I've done a considerable amount of research on death, and what I've come to realize is that for people who are going through this process, one of the biggest things they are distressed about is, "How will I be remembered?"

When my mom was ill, I hired dad to make an iBook of their life together. Mom loved it because it was a legacy of who she was, the impact she had on this world, and it was something for her children and grandchildren to look back on. My Dad liked it so much, he made one for himself. Now that I'm facing a possible shortened timeline, I think about what I'll be remembered by? How do you go about leaving a legacy?

There are so many things I'm passionate about. The world is so connected and, also, troubled because of our inability to disconnect. Yet despite all this, we've lost the capacity to genuinely connect with one another in meaningful and healthy ways. Pay attention when you find yourself in deep meaningful conversations, or an exchange of any kind. Consciously remind yourself of the great thing that's happening, as opposed to just having it happen and moving on.

For example, when I walk out of this coffee shop and ask myself what made our interaction so awesome, the younger Jim would say, "that was a great contact to have for the future." Wiser Jim is aware that this is just a beautiful moment and a great shared experience. Because of my lessons with cancer, I recognize when something good is happening, in the moment. I don't need to know why or where it will go. It makes life so much easier, don't you think?

As a kid, I flipped a car going too fast around a blind corner. I pulled everyone out of the car and as I was waiting for help to arrive, I realized my wrist was broken. In the chaos I felt no pain, similar to when I'm in my cancer pain, I feel less of it because I am present and in the moment. For me, happiness comes through making those I love happy. Then joy just naturally follows me around.

Plus, I've stopped trying to do everything myself, and I listen to my wife's advice on my health. Her role is more powerful than it once was. My role is following her broad-view perspective. I allow her to have more control over my schedule and my health journey. You see, I tend to over-commit. She keeps me grounded and able to manage my life. She understands my inability to say no. I find it easier to be truly happy when you take care of yourself and your family first. That's the beauty of a loving wife and family. They see the whole picture.

Years ago, I used to wait until the family went to bed, and then I'd work on my projects until 1:00 a.m. These days I'm asleep by 10:00. I have competent co-workers and friends around me. They take care of most of the details of my big ideas that I used to manage on my own. And the remarkable thing is, they are finding their own passion in the work. Besides, when you give someone a task to do on their own, they come up with unique solutions. Not to mention, they have the satisfaction of having solved it on their own. It's all getting done. The sooner we learn that we are replaceable, the less stress we take on trying to do it all. It's a win-win.

With all this extra time, I can concentrate on my meditation, visualization, and mindful living. When I'm in the middle of a round of treatment, I make that a priority. I visualize the chemo getting to the centre of my tumour. It's actually turned into a funny thing. I see a magical f*c#ing unicorn doing all the work for me.

Yup, you heard me, a magical f*c#ing unicorn working on the tumour. Excuse the profanity, but you see, unicorns need a little cussing in order to do their best work.

This nonsensical imagery has given me a great deal of comfort I tell myself I am healthy and nothing else. In that moment, I align those cells, and the cells have no choice but to believe in health. Sound a little crazy? Well, I'm still here, so I'm going with crazy.

Part of what I'm trying to do with the tub talks and these awkward conversations is to be known for engaging in the difficult conversations. And you know what? It's going to be really awkward when in ten years I'm still here and the tub talks keep inspiring others. My idea is to do what you need to do to get through it. Don't worry about what others have to say about it.

Go ahead. Fill the bath with bubbles. Share your story. Love those you come in contact with. Stop judging.

And remember my mother's Top Three Things to a Happy Life:

"Be Nice ~ Life is Easy ~ Laugh a Lot"

Blog: GatherWithJim.com

Jim Bits-Tub Talks with Jim & Dave:
https://www.youtube.com/watch?v=Wf1rwRWHSmc

Dave Kelly Live: http://davekellylive.com

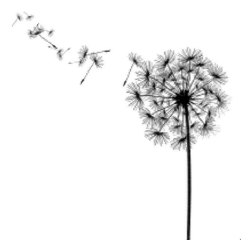

4. Leaving a Legacy

The definition of legacy is often misinterpreted. It's impossible to know what it will look like until you've moved on in this world. They are also largely based on how others perceive you and how you choose to share your experiences. A legacy comes in many forms, with a multitude of meanings. Legacies and are often misinterpreted as an aspect of a business, or to some, are predominately reserved for those of wealth or influence.

When I refer to legacy in this chapter, I see it as a direct result of how we impact the people in our lives while we are living, and in turn how they carry on with our actions, accomplishments or philanthropy after we are gone. Legacy could be to family, friends, colleagues, caregivers, or simply those we interact with on a semi-regular basis.

When I consider the individuals who have impacted me the most, I remember their kindness, compassion, dedication, and tenacity. It's not just a person in a leadership position who has the ability to influence. You make a difference in the lives of others when you are intentional with your interactions when you show up and act with integrity and truth.

I encourage you to write down the people, actions, and conversations that impacted you the most in your life up until this point.

My challenge to those wondering what their legacy will be is to redefine the word. You don't need to reconstruct your entire life, family or community to make a significant impact.

- ✓ Who or what has made a difference in your life and why? The why is a clue here, because it indicates what you value.
- ✓ You make a difference when people walk away from an interaction with you feeling seen and heard.
- ✓ You make a difference when you are unconditionally kind in your words and actions.
- ✓ You impact others when you stand up for what is right even when that means standing alone.
- ✓ You change things when someone says they are better for having known you.

Legacies are formed not only in your substantial actions, but also the countless minuscule actions. When we are intentional about how we show up in our lives and in the lives of others, we set the foundation for remarkable things to happen in the futures of those we leave behind.

Options for leaving a lasting legacy...

Support the People and Causes That Are Close to Your Heart

Jim Button makes family a priority, devoting his time, love and support to his children and wife first. Then Jim includes his extended family, friends, and coworkers. When you are in his company, you know you are the centre of his undivided attention.

Jim is the founder and mastermind behind multiple causes. He supports and cultivates them despite the current health challenges he's facing. When his health forces him to recalibrate his time and energy, he asks for help implementing them.

Honestly and Openly Share Stories with Your Loved Ones

Do an inventory of what's important to you. What has shaped your life? Be an open book. Now is not the time to hold back the truth. Use kindness in your words. Share the funny, the difficult, the challenges, the lessons. Let those you love, know you through the stories of your life.

Give the Gift of Time

Most children, grandchildren, family, and friends remember the gift of time more than they remember monetary gifts. Commit enough of yourself to others, in order that the legacy you leave is based on the fact you loved the people in your life enough to share yourself with them.

Become a Mentor

A mentor, by definition, is a more experienced or more knowledgeable person in an area of expertise. Everyone has a significant truth to impart to others that will guide and inspire.

In chapter 9 Charlie Scopoletti shares his music with the world. Physical discomfort disappears when he shares this experience.

Chapter 5 reveals how Tim Ding became a mentor to cancer

patients. He believes it to be one of the reasons he's alive today. In giving his time and wisdom to others, his health prospers.

Barbara Marx Hubbard developed a program to teach others how to redefine the role of illness in upcoming chapter 11.

Jim Button spends time in a bubble bath with a friend, mentoring through humour and honesty.

While reading chapter 7 you discover how Luisa shares her smile and is mentoring a new generation of children on the simple beauty of sharing happiness.

Jen Gardiner opened her heart to love and taught others the value of embracing love, giving love, and receiving love in chapter 1.

Pursue What Makes You Happy – Happiness Turns into a Passion

When you find what makes you truly happy, it has the gift of passions intricately woven within it, and then that passion can become your legacy. Happiness and/or passion comes from a wellspring of the intentions, interests, and beliefs you've lived. Finding and cultivating that happiness allows you to see your destiny ahead of time. It's contagious for every person with whom you come in contact.

Charlie Scopoletti found that happiness comes from writing and performing his music. His life passion comes in the form of words, lyrics, and music. Inspiring others has turned into the healing effects that music provides, not only to himself but to countless others around the globe.

When an idea comes to you that feels like fun, pursue it. Never stop searching for or sharing your happiness. Happy thoughts find and attract more of the same. Isn't that a lovely thought!

Leaving a legacy is an important part of your life's mission. Legacies are born from passion, and passion is interconnected to emotions such as happiness, bliss, contentment delight, glee, and laughter.

Jim Button writes a blog to share his passion for open, honest dialogue. That may not be your outlet but consider a time or a place where you have an opportunity to share a simple smile. You never know what heart that smile will land on. It may be received by someone who needs it more than you realize. And it's free to give.

What is it you imagine people will write about you when you're gone? What story are you living that will continue? These are questions to consider about what kind of legacy your current life will leave. If you don't like how that story is unfolding, change it. If all you can do is share wisdom, share your wisdom with those who'll listen. Improving the life of one person is more than enough of a legacy...

Write it down

Not a writer? No problem. Share your life story by way of a recording device, your phone, video or computer. Borrow one if need be. The great thing about your voice is it's personal to you, and the families love to hear you speak. Especially after you're gone. That might be in a month or fifty years' time. Keep telling your stories and sharing the wisdom you've acquired. Age is not a prerequisite for wisdom or storytelling. Listening to a child, a teenager, grandparent or neighbour is a precious gift that is free to give. Write their words down and share them with others. It is how legacies are built, one word, one story, one lesson at a time.

What is it you plan to do with your one wild and precious life?

Mary Oliver wrote; *The Summer Day* in 1992. In Oliver's brilliantly simple yet complex poem, she poses the question: *what is it you plan to do with this one wild and precious life?* Her words speak of the simple moments that make up each one of our lives. We have seconds, minutes, hours, days and years. But we never know exactly when they will end.

In chapter one, Jen Gardiner spoke of the fact she was given a timeline of two years to live. She decided then and there to make them the most spectacular two years of her life. Deciding that she would not miss anything, by living the remainder of her time on earth with joy and curiosity. Jen called her cancer diagnosis a time when her *living clock* started counting down. She did everything in her power to make life joyous, sharing the most ridiculous and the most subtle of moments with those she loved. What became vital to her was to share her life, however long it turned out to be. Quality was now the goal in her one wild and precious life.

What do you want for your one wild and precious life? I'm inviting you to choose yours. With or without a living clock counting down.

The Summer Day

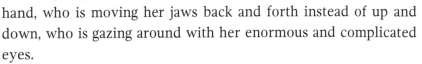

Who made the world?

Who made the swan, and the
black bear?

Who made the grasshopper?

This grasshopper, I mean,
the one who has flung herself
out of the grass, the one who
is eating sugar out of my
hand, who is moving her jaws back and forth instead of up and
down, who is gazing around with her enormous and complicated
eyes.

Now she lifts her pale forearms and thoroughly washes her face.

Now she snaps her wings open and floats away. I don't know
exactly what a prayer is.

I do know how to pay attention, how to fall down into the grass,
how to kneel down in the grass, how to be idle and blessed, how to
stroll through the fields, which is what I have been doing all day.

Tell me, what else should I have done? Doesn't everything die at
last, and too soon?

Tell me, what is it you plan to do with your one wild and precious
life?

By Mary Oliver

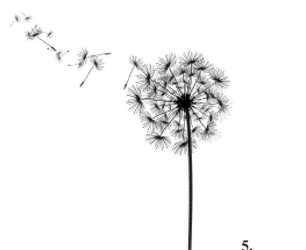

5.   **Tim Ding**

How Cancer Saved My Life

Tim Ding has a zest and appreciation for life that's expressed through his soulful eyes, affectionate smile, and contagious laugh. Joy, acceptance, and compassion flow freely from his very being.

I asked him what he preferred to be called, Tim or Timothy, and his answer set the tone for the interview: "Whatever is comfortable on your lips." Tim's cancer was discovered during a yearly check-up in the summer of 2000. In this chapter, Tim reveals how an unexpected community transformed his experience and saved him from himself.

Tim Ding

My doctor discovered a very small cyst on my kidney through an ultrasound test. It was decided a keyhole surgery two weeks later would be used to remove it. During the surgery, it became evident that a second surgery was required to remove the left kidney because the tiny cyst the had grown to the size of a small Coke-Cola bottle.

One week of waiting for the biopsy results turned into three, and my cancer journey began with the news that not only did I have kidney cancer, but I was also the first kidney cancer patient in Singapore; not exactly an honour worthy of celebration.

I'm a person who values my privacy. I made the choice to only share the news with my wife, parents, and siblings. I honestly didn't believe people cared, nor did I want sympathy from friends or coworkers, or worse yet, strangers offering hollow prayers for me. But five operations later, a host of complications, infections, chemotherapy, a lengthy roadmap of stitches, had left me bedridden and incapable of sitting up or caring for myself, let alone my family. The prognosis was bleak. What was so vital to begin with, – my privacy, – became an obstacle as the repercussion of cancer and its treatments revealed themselves.

When you find yourself at the end of a rope, you hold on with one hand and search for a lifeline with the other. That lifeline came in the form of a community I wasn't aware existed, it consisted of a group of Catholic women in my neighbourhood. They somehow heard about my health crisis and approached my wife saying they'd designed a program, a timetable of sorts, where they would come to our home and help with food, cleaning and caring for me. If I agreed, my wife could go to work, and they would look after the details of home-life. My wife wouldn't have the added stress of working, caring for the household, and her bedridden husband.

My secret was out; the lifeline I was searching for required I relinquish my privacy and allow strangers to help my family. Strangers from a religious institution I didn't believe in. Strangers taking care of me. Strangers who – I suspected – would be praying for me. Funny thing is, the renouncement of my freedom, was as difficult to accept as my illness.

I had no choice but to surrender my pride and accept the help of others. When they came to our home, they said to me, "Relax: if you need anything, ring the bell, or shout out." They not only helped me, but they also offered assistance to my ailing father. I think they were saying prayers for me in the other room, however, they never openly prayed in front of me. They knew I was a non-believer and that didn't matter to them; they came to help a family in their time of need, not a belief system.

In my vulnerable state, those women taught me about caring, giving, how to listen, and faith. Not faith in a church or a dogma, they communicated through selfless acts: they gave of themselves with no expectations of reward or recognition. To my surprise, I found myself praying. I'm not sure why because I'm not a religious man. I didn't know Bible verses, nor did I have the first-hand experience with praying.

As unlikely as it seems now, I literally began my journey in prayer, with a long list of complaints to God. I was the poorest example of a testimony to faith that you could ever imagine. I was angry with life, pain, death, cancer, and I was desperate for answers:

- ✓ *"This is not fair, there are so many things that I haven't done."*
- ✓ *"I want to do so many things!"*
- ✓ *"I really don't care about your salvation."*
- ✓ *"I don't care about your Heaven or Hell."*

I came to God in such a raw and troubled way. I prayed the only way I knew how: through dispute and bargains. I'd shut the world out of my life, but through the kindness of strangers, I found an open door that led directly to my heart.

I started talking to God every day. I'd say: *"God are you there? I need to discuss some things with you because, well, you are God, right?"* In my conversation with him I reasoned, *"I'd better let you be God and I'll be man,"* – and for the first time, I let God be God. Even a non-Christian like myself understood that: it's a good idea to respect God because he is a higher being. He can't be *seen*, but he can be felt.

And so, I began to reason with him: *"Seriously, this is so unfair. God, I have a beautiful wife who is too young to be a widow and a precious one-year-old daughter who needs her father. My aging parents are too old to care for themselves with me gone. It's not fair to these four people."* I rationalized: *"I'm a hopeless case; it's logical for you to take me, but it's not fair to my family that I die at this point, I need you to make sense of this."*

This was how my conversations with God began. I believe if you speak honestly and in your own words, the patterns and structure of the sentences don't matter. There are times when I felt like a Buddhist in Zen meditation because when I had no words for him, I'd sit in his presence and say, *"God I don't know what to tell you today; I have mood swings because of the chemotherapy, my emotions are not good right now. Please bear with me if I speak with any sin before you. I may be uttering nonsense, but then you are God, you understand. I must remember that."*

All the prayers and treatments failed to produce the results I'd hoped for, and eventually, I found myself face to face with my doctor asking the tough question:

"How much time do I have?" He reluctantly replied, "Nine months."

Not surprisingly, after a 'death row' sentence, I had a long list of questions for my doctor, and the most urgent to me was, "How do I live these remaining 270 days: carefully, or wildly?

I'd become so obedient to the cancer, that my life became not so much living as it was serving my illness. My Doctor's answer surprised me,

"Tim, you have nine months to live. Do what you want. Eat what you want. Live life on your terms, just don't hurt yourself or others. Do whatever it is YOU WANT TO DO."

With no further treatment options available; his final prescription for me was to live these remaining 270 days my way. With that, he set me free from the restrictive protocol of a terminal illness. It was up to me, not cancer, to decide how I would live the time I had left.

I thought of the last moments I would have with my daughter, my wife, family, and friends. My last Christmas, last Chinese New Year, last springtime. I had nine months of endings; I could choose to live them *opening up or closing down.* My heart urged me in the direction of joy. I read somewhere that the definition of joy is "happy, for no reason."

Eventually, my external wounds healed and through the example of the community that formed to support me, I discovered a need to tear down the walls around my heart in relation to spirituality. Through these ongoing conversations I was having with the God I came to know; I stumbled my way into a new passion. I found myself turning in the direction of giving back to the cancer community.

A journey of this nature is unique to us all: God, Infinite, Buddha, Divine, Jesus, Mohammed, Allah, Universe, Spirit – the name or process doesn't matter. It came to me in a way that worked for me: not by reciting Bible verses, confessing my sins, or repeating specific prayers. I realized God is the little voice in my heart and through these conversations, I found my way, inside. At first, it's an experience of you listening to yourself: once you get past your own thoughts and stop believing them, you begin to realize there are answers within that you need to know.

The God I know is not restrictive. He would not give me, a staunch non-believer, the Ten Commandments: thou shall not do this – thou shall not do that. The God I came to know, mirrored what the doctor said: "Go out there and do whatever you want, just don't hurt people or yourself." I released my resistance to all the things I was holding on to that didn't serve me, and I did just that. And guess what, it was then that my life and the lives of everyone around me improved. No one is ever hurt or disrespected. Today, I live with purpose, and it makes sense to me. My wife will never understand the new level of relationship I have with God, but as long as I'm not hurting her or anyone else, she accepts my choices.

Our lives are richer in every way.

Those who have never walked my walk could be convinced that I'm making all this up or attempting to console myself with something that can't be proven. I believe there is power in the affirmation, *Let God be God*, but I also believe in allowing every-one to walk along their own path. For me, these conversations are like a meditation: I listen to my heart and it's overflowing with answers, and not just for me. I speak to my God and say, *"I'm going to visit this cancer patient today, what should I tell him?"* The answer is always the same: *"Just go and have fun, tell them whatever you like, what you think is proper."* You see, the advice I get for other people is the same as for me: have fun, don't hurt anyone and do what you think is right. It's not complicated and it's the same for all of us.

On Good Friday, I was watching TV and they were showing *The Passion of The Christ*. It was probably the tenth time it was playing because every TV station here in Singapore loves to screen it. I suddenly had a thought in my head. This inner voice came into my head and said, *"Hey if someone was coming to your house, what would you do?"* I responded, *"Well, I would clean up my house. Make my house tidy and invite the guests into a clean home and make them feel comfortable and welcome."* And this voice said, *"How many times do you make an effort to clean up your heart? I've been sitting here in your heart, but you have not been cleaning up anything."* My response was a resounding, *"It's time for spring cleaning."* I decided I would do some inner spring cleaning.

Since that time, I've discovered this is a progressive practice; it takes time. I'm not any more or less special, than the next person. I made the decision to listen to my heart. I tell cancer patients all the time: if you sit quietly and listen to your heart, you will hear your inner voice. It has wisdom for you if you are willing to listen.

I had a blank piece of paper right before me, and I started writing, *"Cancer did not happen because I acted poorly, and my renewed health did not happen because I got in touch with God. These changes happened because I let God be God."*

I think God touched my heart somewhere in the night, not because I'm any more special than another, but because I'm open.

Suddenly it hit me that there are a lot more things involved than just me wanting to live the life I want.

Life is precious. I can do all that I want but living that way can be quite selfish – it can be done in a very selfish manner. I looked at my anger and I realized that was a selfish act and it got me thinking, this is not just about inner spring cleaning, it's about cancer patients having so many things in their heart. I think God revealed this in a very supernatural way to me in order to help people who are suffering from an illness, and in particular, cancer patients. But really, it's no different for us all. What became clear to me was that it would be better to release all the hurt and the pain in our hearts. What's the point of keeping all that hurt inside, and a better question is what damage is it doing to you holding on to it?

As a cancer patient, our wishes and dreams are immediate. We have endless questions without answers, long To-Do lists we may never realize. You want to do it all, and often we become scattered in one area and over-focused in another. I became preoccupied with my family and love. What I learned is that we all have an immense capacity to love. More importantly, to love one another is to love yourself and you can't love somebody unless you find what it is you love about yourself. I believe most people are taught to go out and find love outside themselves. The truth I've come to know is:

Love is at the core of your heart and your happiness. You need to look within before you EVER find it in a person, place or possession.

Initially, I believed it was OK for me to have cancer because I was flawed. I had convinced myself that my family was better than me and they deserve the best possible life. It wasn't until I started loving and honouring myself that I came to understand how I was holding back love. I had to stop judging myself as undeserving of love or I would never find true love or peace. Not just in my body and mind, but in my relationships too. I didn't have a relationship with the Infinite before my cancer. I didn't want one. Something changed inside of me when I engaged in conversations from deep within my heart. I started to hear – not with my ears, I began to hear with my heart.

In order to be whole, it's necessary to love and honour the exceptional AND the unacceptable aspects of who you are. Learn how to look at your bones, your kidneys, liver, brain, eyes, feet, and fingernails; love all of you, unconditionally.

Lavish yourself with quality food, the best shampoo, nail polish, and personal care products that you can afford. Treat yourself with the respect you would give someone you were head over heels in love with. When you feel respected and loved inside, you are able to give and receive love in return.

After learning how to love myself, I discovered an immense capacity to give. I searched out a community of cancer patients who needed my help. I spent time with them, shared my experience, actively listened to their fears and dreams, or simply held their hand and said a silent prayer. I offered them what the community of women gave me: love, respect, non-judgment, listening, and time. I encouraged them to look in the corner of their heart: it's there that their higher self awaits them – waiting to talk, willing to listen. I wanted them to find comfort and self-acceptance.

I have sat with many cancer patients who have since healed and I've sat with an equal amount who've passed away. Many who come to a peaceful death and many who do not. I don't judge their body's choice to die. I learn from them and hopefully, they learn from me. It seems strange to not feel sad when someone dies, but it's in helping them die with love and free from fear that keeps me going back. I'm equally happy when I help someone live, as when I help them die. I've learned that living and dying are agreements we make when we are born. I believe it's through honouring yourself in every way, it's there that you find peace when your lifeline is drawing to a close.

After receiving a terminal diagnosis, you count every day and when the nine-month mark arrived, I called the doctor and said, "Hey, I'm still kicking, I'm alive." He told me to come back as he wanted to have a look at me one more time. Medically he couldn't understand why I survived, but he told me to keep doing whatever it was I was doing. I agreed and dutifully listened to the prescription of my heart. Even though the doctor was closely monitoring my progress, it wasn't until I reached the five-year mark that he sat me down to ask exactly what protocol I was following in all areas of my life. I told him that something switched inside me when I started to treat myself with absolute respect.

When I sit down to eat nutritious food, I'd thank God and pray the food would nourish me better than the medicine the doctors were giving me. I was grateful in all areas of my life. I couldn't be kind and understanding to the patients I sat with at the hospital if I wasn't respecting myself: my body, my mind, and my soul. It was as much a gift to them as it was for me. The by-product of basic respect for myself evolved into reverence for everything and everyone.

I told him I was volunteering my time and experience with cancer patients. That I was following his prescription of doing what I wanted respecting others was a vital key, yet I was also living my life on my terms; doing what was best for me. It sounds selfish, but why would we not treat ourselves with the kindness and love we want in return? It's impossible to give absolute love and respect to others when you don't have it within yourself.

My doctor had the pleasure of clearing me medically. He defined the reason for my healing as a positive mental attitude. I said, "I don't know about that, but I think that I am having a great relationship now and this relationship is with a higher power. It can't be tested or measured because it has no limits or borders. It's infinite." I learned firsthand about giving absolute love and respect from the community of women who came into my home. They never pushed their religion on me, and it was a good thing because I had no traditional experience with the infinite. I was angry with my situation, I needed to find the path that best suited me. Through the example of giving without expectation or judgment, what grew inside of me was the deep desire to give back.

I believe giving is a direct route to receiving what you need. When my body was healthy enough, I found a growing desire to sit with others giving back what I'd been given; love, respect, time and a complete lack of judgment.

For me to be able to give back to other cancer patients, I must first have a real experience that I am talking to God as himself. I don't know the kind of process a religious person follows – the God, I've come to know, is able to listen to me sensibly. I find that when I first began to talk to the Infinite, I needed to be sensible inside. Many of today's religious teachings try to sell God; they treat the Infinite so cheaply. If you talk to God and you don't let God be God, you had better wash your lips. I think He's extremely private; He doesn't gossip, He never tells you what to do. You can trust Him.

I think one of the ways I came out of cancer was because I started telling God everything in my heart. The good things and the bad things too. Really, the measurement of bad and good comes from the judgemental view of another person, it comes from whether *they* believe something is good or bad. God doesn't judge if something is wrong or right, he asks you to experience it for yourself. He says, "Do it and see how you feel about it. If this rubs against you...don't do it. If it caresses you...do it, and then just enjoy yourself."

What caresses me is to visit cancer patients on a volunteer basis. People message me asking, "Could you pray for so and so?" and I just go and visit, and it makes me feel happy. I find more of these cancer patients experiencing some relief in their cancer.

There are those who ask me to sit and listen while they talk to whoever they believe in, and they just let go of everything. We cry for hours, and after that, I see only peace on their face. At first, they say, "this isn't working out at all' and then they just start living. So, you see, you continue dying, or you start living. They start to live, and they suddenly stop dying. Then they tell their friends. In the Bible, it says Jesus tells his followers before he goes into the heavens that they are to go into the world to teach the gospel and make disciples.

Well, I think that making disciples is not a structured program where you need to have a degree in Bible studies. I think that making disciples is to show people the way: to find peace first with yourself and let God be God in your heart. I think most people today are taught how to ask God to do something. I think in my journey it is that I say, "God you are there, you do what you want. I just have to talk with you." I have never known a God who was demanding me to go to the missions of India; that has never been my experience with the Infinite, and it's served me well, I'm still around to talk about it today. I think there is a God. So that's how I get along in my life. I still count on my calendar, but not to the day I die, rather I count how many days I have been blessed from the day I was diagnosed. My surgeon gave me nine months to live; that was nineteen years ago and counting.

Cancer saved my life by waking me up to the world around me. I'm never alone on this path unless I choose to be alone.

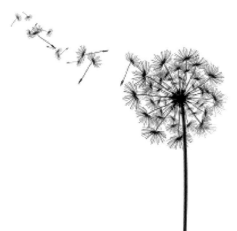

6. Communities Listen

Tim Ding recounted his experience with community. He was a private and solitary – family man whose only wish was to care for his family. Following a diagnosis of cancer and the debilitating surgeries that followed, he found himself incapacitated and unable to care for either his family or himself. Word spread throughout the area he lived in and a community of women came to his rescue.

Here was a proud, non-religious man in need of help and the people who came to his rescue were a group of Catholic women who, in addition to helping him physically, were secretly praying for him in another room. They cared for him while his body healed and in the quiet moments of desperation, he came to terms with a previously non-existent relationship to spirituality and a community that appeared when he found himself at the end of his ever-fraying rope.

What is the definition of community? The Webster dictionary describes community as; "a unified body of individuals: people with common interests; a group of people with a common characteristic or interest living together within a larger society."

My belief and definition of community encompass a slightly broader perspective. I believe a community can be almost anyone and anywhere that we are in relation to another human or living being. A community can be as small as two, or as expansive as an entire nation. As Tim convalesced in his room, a compassionate group of spiritual women, he once felt had no connection to him, prayed and cared for him free of the need for him to believe in a higher power or for that matter to even participate.

What began as an outreach of helping hands transformed Tim Ding into an avid community man with a voracious appetite for giving back to the cancer community of which he reluctantly found himself a part of. Community and Volunteerism turned this intensely private family man into a patient listener and dedicated advocate of the power of prayer and community.

What makes community such a powerful healing force? In our hurry-up world, we've moved away from the once normal practice of living in communities to the privacy of the modern-day living. We live in single-family homes or apartments and we draw our shades and lock the doors. We travel to work alone, eat our meals in chosen groups or isolated. We exercise by ourselves, often connected to music to keep others from interacting. Spontaneity is a thing of the past. We even make appointments to drop in on friends or text to see if it's ok to call. There are days when human connection is reduced to keystrokes on a keyboard. We proudly call this progress, yet we've become sicker, with higher rates of depression and we are lonelier than we've ever been in history. Our modern lifestyle of seeking to be alone has devastating effects on our mental, spiritual and physical health.

A study has been going on for 58+ years in the close-knit group of Italian immigrants living in a Pennsylvania community. It's been dubbed, *The Roseto Effect*. The study was initiated as a way to discover why, in the early 60s, the people living in Roseto, Pennsylvania had such a low incidence of heart attacks. As the study progressed, researchers discovered that this group of Italian immigrants had a mortality rate uncommonly low for the United States. Within ten years of the start of the study, an unexpected and deadly virus infected the community and the findings became of intense interest to more than just the researchers. The world took note of *The Roseto Effect*.

What was different in the beautiful and remarkably modest town of Roseto nestled in Eastern Pennsylvania? For 200 years, togetherness was second nature to these Italian immigrants who had come from Italy to settle in Roseto in 1882. The inhabitants were hard-working, healthy, interconnected, youthful, vital and joyful. In 1961, in what would prove to be a landmark study named after the town, *The Roseto Effect*, made its mark. A group of researchers descended on Roseto with all the equipment of scientific investigators...and with the blessings of the Federal and State governments, this town became the center of interest. There was talk that this little town was the fountain of youth. Why? Because Roseto was a distinctly healthier place to live according to statistics. Researchers were determined to find out why!

The Rosetans were poked, prodded, questioned, studied and compared to neighbouring communities. The unusually low mortality rate continued to be confirmed with every aspect investigated. And the conclusions have had tremendous implications even now.

Let's go back to the 1960s. If you were to visit the small town of Roseto, you would have witnessed local men returning from gruelling days spent in notoriously toxic slate-quarries. The women would be returning home from the blouse sewing factory, where they laboured in order to send their children to college (which they did at a rate far above the national average). You would find the Rosetans strolling along the village's main street as they stopped to chat with neighbours who were resting on chairs outside their front doors. They would most likely share a glass of wine before heading home to wash and change for dinner.

Each evening the local women would gather together in communal kitchens to prepare classic Italian dishes. Unlike today's Mediterranean diet consisting of olive oil, salads and fat-free foods, the Rosetans, unable to afford imported olive oil, fried their sausages, and meatballs in heavy lard. They ate prosciutto and salami that was paired with hard and soft cheeses, not to mention the usual glass or two of homemade red wine.

While the mammas cooked dinner, the children entertained themselves by playing soccer, climbing trees, or running freely in the town square. In between visiting and smoking their cigars, men pushed tables together in anticipation of the nightly ritual that gathered the community over heaping piles of pasta, homemade sauce, meat, and free-flowing vino. Conversations were filled with laughter, political discussion, advice on family issues and the planning of upcoming celebrations. It seemed that those overflowing dinner tables offered nourishment for the human spirit as well as the body. In was becoming clear to the researchers that the communal rituals consisting of the evening stroll, the numerous clubs, church festivals, birthdays and neighbourhood gatherings that included the whole community coming together, contributed to the villagers' good health.

The residents of Roseto made it their business to look out for one another. Multi-generational homes were the norm, families cared for families as well as neighbours. Monday to Friday, villagers went to the same workplace and on Sundays, they all went to church together. Neighbours wandered in and out of each other's kitchens and holidays were joyously celebrated communally.

The individual residents of Roseto were never left to struggle through life alone, no one was lonely because you were part of a greater family, no matter your age or social standing. Roseto was living proof: the power of community keeps you healthy. They smoked old-style Italian cigars, drank wine every night; in fact, wine was preferred over soft drinks and even milk. Despite these seemingly unhealthy food choices, the residents of Roseto risk of heart attack deaths were half the national average. As the study progressed, researchers discovered an uncommonly low instance of depression and common viruses. Each house studied contained three families or three generations. The elderly were neither institutionalized nor marginalized, they were revered and respected, the villages looked up to them as informal judges and arbitrators in everyday life and commerce. Residents were healthy not because of genetics, better doctors, exercise, or something in their water supply. They appeared to be immunized by the collaborative oneness of community.

Rosetans, regardless of income and education, expressed them-selves in a family-centered social life. There was a total absence of ostentation among the wealthy; those who had more money didn't flaunt it. There was nearly exclusive patronage of local businesses, even with bigger shops and stores in nearby towns. The Italians from regional cities in Italy intermarried in Roseto, the families were close-knit, self-supportive and independent, but also relied especially in bad times on the greater community for well-defined assistance and friendly help. Researchers ultimately concluded that love, intimacy and being part of a community protected their health.

John Bruhn, a sociologist, and author of The Power of Clan writes about The Roseto Effect. He recalls, *"There was no suicide, no alcoholism, no drug addiction, and very little crime. They didn't have anyone on welfare. Then we looked at peptic ulcers. They didn't have any of those either. These people were dying of old age. That's it."*

Then Everything Changed...

As time went on, the younger generation was less charmed by life in Roseto. To them, it seemed immune to modernization.

When the young people went off to study at college, they brought back to Roseto new ideas, new dreams, and new people. Italian Americans started marrying non-Italians. The children strayed from the church, joined country clubs, and moved into single-family suburban houses with fences and pools.

With these changes, the multi-generational homes disbanded and the community lifestyle shifted gears from nightly celebrations to more of the typical, every man for himself philosophy of today. The neighbours who would regularly drop in for casual visits started phoning each other to schedule appointments. The evening rituals of adults singing songs while children played soccer in the square turned into nights in front of the television, segregated from the community.

In 1971, when heart attack rates in other parts of the country were dropping because of widespread adoption of healthier diets and regular exercise programs, Roseto had its first heart attack death in someone younger than 45. Over the next decade, heart disease rates in Roseto doubled. The incidence of high blood pressure tripled. The number of strokes increased. Sadly, by 1979, the number of fatal heart attacks in Roseto had increased to the national average.

As it turns out, human beings nourish each other by being together, and the health of the body reflects this. Rosetans gave up their intimate contact with a loving community and it cost them their health.

In the book, *The Power of Clan*, co-authors John Bruhn and Stewart Wolf covered the Roseto Study from 1935-1984 Their conclusions dovetailed with the other studies.

"The magic of Roseto was the total avoidance of isolated individuals crushed by problems of everyday life. Rosetans didn't feel isolated or crushed, rather they avoided the internalization of stress. Stability and predictability – hardly Americanized virtues – even in the early years, life was soothing, hence life-lengthening."

In chapter 5, when Tim Ding found himself in a new and unwanted community after his cancer surgery, he resisted and suffered emotionally because he believed being alone was in his best interest. His wife had to work to support the family and he couldn't take care of his physical needs. A further insult was when a religious group of women who were strangers, stepped in to help.

For Tim, the very fact, they were associated with a spiritual group annoyed him. He believed they were trying to convert him to find God. Years later with his health restored, Tim Ding became a volunteer and community leader. He believes that *finding a community and learning how to listen to himself and others*, are two of the reasons he's alive.

How can you implement these two lessons: Community and Active Listening that Tim believes saved him?

Let's start with a few ideas on *Volunteering* by Jeanne Segal, Ph.D. and Lawrence Robinson

Why Volunteer?

Volunteering offers vital help to people in need, to worthwhile causes, and to the community, but the benefits can be even greater for you, the volunteer. Volunteering and helping others can help you reduce stress, combat depression, keep you mentally stimulated, and provide a sense of purpose. While it's true that the more you volunteer, the more benefits you'll experience, volunteering doesn't have to involve a long-term commitment or take a huge amount of time out of your busy day. Giving, even in simple ways can help those in need and improve your health and happiness.

Volunteering: The Happiness Effect

Benefits of volunteering to feel healthier and happier
- ✓ Volunteering connects you to others
- ✓ Volunteering is good for your mind and body
- ✓ Volunteering can advance your career
- ✓ Volunteering brings fun and fulfillment to your life

Benefit 1: Volunteering connects you to others

One of the better-known benefits of volunteering is the impact on the community. Volunteering allows you to connect to your community and make it a better place. Helping out with even the smallest tasks can make a real difference to the lives of people, animals, and organizations in need. And volunteering is a two-way street: it can benefit you and your family as much as it benefits the cause you choose to help. Dedicating your time as a volunteer helps you make new friends, expand your network, and boost your social skills.

Make new friends and contacts

One of the best ways to make new friends and strengthen existing relationships is to commit to a shared activity together. Volunteering is a great way to meet new people, especially if you are new to an area. It strengthens your ties to the community and broadens your support network, exposing you to people with common interests, neighbourhood resources, fun and fulfilling activities.

Increase your social and relationship skills

While some people are naturally outgoing, others are shy and have a hard time meeting new people. Volunteering gives you the opportunity to practice and develop your social skills since you are meeting regularly with a group of people with common interests. Once you have momentum, it's easier to branch out and make more friends and contacts.

Volunteering as a family

Children watch everything you do. By giving back to the community, you teach them firsthand how volunteering makes a difference. They learn how good it feels to help other people and animals, and how to enact change. It's also a valuable way for you to get to know organizations in the community and find resources and activities for your children and family.

Benefit 2: Volunteering is good for your mind and body

Volunteering provides many benefits to both mental and physical health. Volunteering helps counteract the effects of stress, anger, and anxiety. The social contact aspect of helping and working with others can have a profound effect on your overall psychological wellbeing.

Nothing relieves stress better than a meaningful connection to another person. Working with pets and other animals have also been shown to improve mood and reduce stress and anxiety.

Volunteering combats depression

Volunteering keeps you in regular contact with others and helps you develop a solid support system, which, in turn protects, you against depression.

Volunteering makes you happy. By measuring hormones and brain activity, researchers have discovered that being helpful to others delivers immense pleasure. Human beings are hardwired to give to others. The more we give, the happier we feel.

Volunteering increases self-confidence. You are doing good for others and the community, which provides a natural sense of accomplishment. Your role as a volunteer can also give you a sense of pride and identity. And the better you feel about yourself, the more likely you are to have a positive view of your life and future goals.

Volunteering provides a sense of purpose

Older adults, especially those who have retired or lost a spouse, can find new meaning and direction in their lives by helping others. Whatever your age or life situation, volunteering can help take your mind off your own worries, keep you mentally stimulated, and add more zest to your life.

Volunteering helps you stay physically healthy. Studies have found that those who volunteer have a lower mortality rate than those who do not.

Older volunteers tend to walk more, find it easier to cope with everyday tasks, are less likely to develop high blood pressure, and have better-thinking skills. Volunteering can also lessen symptoms of chronic pain and reduce the risk of heart disease.

Can I still volunteer, with limited mobility?

People with disabilities or chronic health conditions can still benefit greatly from volunteering. In fact, research has shown that adults with disabilities or health conditions ranging from hearing and vision loss to heart disease, diabetes or digestive disorders all show improvement after volunteering.

Whether due to a disability, a lack of transportation, or time constraints, many people choose to volunteer their time via phone or computer. In today's digital age many organizations need help with writing, graphic design, email, and other web-based tasks. Some organizations may require you to attend an initial training session or periodic meetings, while others can all be done remotely. In any volunteer situation, make sure that you are getting enough social contact, and that the organization is available to support you should you have questions.

Benefit 3: Volunteering can advance your career

If you're considering a new career, volunteering can help you get experience in your area of interest and meet people in the field. Even if you're not planning on changing careers, volunteering gives you the opportunity to practice important skills used in the workplace, such as teamwork, communication, problem-solving, project planning, task management, and organization. You might feel more comfortable stretching your wings at work once you've first honed these skills in a volunteer position first.

Gaining career experience

Volunteering offers you the chance to try out a new career without making a long-term commitment. It is also a great way to gain experience in a new field. In some fields, you can volunteer directly at an organization that does the kind of work you're interested in. If you're interested in nursing, volunteer at a hospital or a nursing home.

Your volunteer work might also expose you to professional organizations or internships that could be of benefit to your career.

Teaching you valuable job skills

Just because volunteer work is unpaid does not mean the skills you learn are only basic. Many volunteering opportunities provide extensive training. You could become an experienced crisis counsellor while volunteering for a women's shelter, or a knowledgeable art historian while donating your time as a museum docent.

Volunteering can also help you build upon skills you already have and use them to benefit the greater community. For instance, if you hold a successful sales position, you can raise awareness for your favourite cause as a volunteer advocate, while further developing and improving your public speaking, communication, and marketing skills.

When it comes to volunteering passion and positivity are the only requirements.

While learning new skills can be beneficial to many, it's not a requirement for a fulfilling volunteer experience. Bear in mind that the most valuable skills you can bring to any volunteer effort are compassion, an open mind, a willingness to do whatever is needed, and a positive attitude.

Benefit 4: Volunteering brings fun and fulfillment to your life

Volunteering is a fun and easy way to explore your interests and passions. Doing volunteer work, you find meaningful and interesting can be a relaxing, energizing escape from your day-to-day routine of work, school, or family commitments. Volunteering also provides you with renewed creativity, motivation, and vision that can carry over into your personal and professional life.

Many people volunteer in order to make time for hobbies outside of work as well. For instance, if you have a desk job and long to spend time outdoors, you might consider volunteering to help plant a community garden, walk dogs for an animal shelter, or help out at a children's camp.

Consider your goals and interests

You will have a richer and more enjoyable volunteering experience if you first take some time to identify your goals and interests. Think about why you want to volunteer. What would you enjoy doing? The opportunities that match both your goals and your interests are most likely to be fun and fulfilling.

Tips for getting started:

First, ask yourself if there is something specific you want to do.

For example, do I want...
- ✓ to make my neighbourhood a better place to live
- ✓ to meet people who are different from me
- ✓ to try something new

- ✓ to do something with my spare time
- ✓ to see a different way of life and new places
- ✓ to have a go at the type of work I might want to do as a full-time job
- ✓ to do more with my interests and hobbies
- ✓ to do something I'm good at

The best way to volunteer is to match your personality and interests.

Having answers to these questions will help you narrow down your search.

The best way to volunteer is to match your personality and interests.

There are numerous volunteer opportunities available. The key is to find a volunteer position that you would enjoy and are capable of doing. It's also important to make sure that your commitment matches the organization's needs. Ask yourself the following:

- ✓ Would you like to work with adults, children, animals, or remotely from home?
- ✓ Do you prefer to work alone or as part of a team?
- ✓ Are you better behind the scenes or do you prefer to take a more visible role?
- ✓ How much time are you willing to commit?
- ✓ What skills can you bring to a volunteer job?
- ✓ What causes are important to you?

Don't limit yourself to just one organization or one specific type of job. Sometimes an opportunity looks great on paper, but the reality is quite different. Try to visit different organizations and get a feel for what they are like and if you click with other staff and volunteers.

Where to find volunteer opportunities

- ✓ Community theatres, museums, and monuments
- ✓ Libraries or senior centres
- ✓ Service organizations such as Lions Clubs or Rotary Clubs
- ✓ Local animal shelters, rescue organizations, or wildlife centres
- ✓ Youth organizations, sports teams, and after-school Programs
- ✓ Historical restorations, national parks, and conservation organizations
- ✓ Places of worship such as churches or synagogues
- ✓ Online databases such as those contained in the resources section below

How much time should you volunteer?

Volunteering doesn't have to take over your life to be beneficial. In fact, research shows that just two to three hours per week, or about 100 hours a year, can offer the most benefits – to both you and your chosen cause. The important thing is to volunteer only the amount of time that feels comfortable to you. Volunteering should feel like a fun and rewarding hobby, not another chore on your to-do list.

Getting the most out of volunteering

You're donating your valuable time, so it's important that you enjoy and benefit from your volunteering. To make sure that your volunteer position is a good fit:

Ask questions

You want to make sure that the experience is right for your skills, your goals, and the time you want to spend. Sample questions to your volunteer coordinator might address your time commitment, whether there's any training involved, who you will be working with, and what to do if you have questions during your experience.

Make sure you know what's expected

You should be comfortable with the organization and understand the time commitment. Consider starting small so that you don't over commit yourself at first. Give yourself some flexibility to change your focus if needed.

Don't be afraid to make a change

Don't force yourself into a bad fit or feel compelled to stick with a volunteer role you dislike. Talk to the organization about changing your focus or look for a different organization that's a better fit.

If volunteering overseas, choose carefully

Some volunteer programs abroad can cause more harm than good if they take much-needed paying jobs away from local workers. Look for volunteer opportunities with reputable organizations.

Enjoy yourself

The best volunteer experiences benefit both the volunteer and the organization. If you're not enjoying yourself, ask yourself why. Is it the tasks you're performing? The people you're working with? Or are you uncomfortable simply because the situation is new and unfamiliar? Pinpointing what's bothering you can help you decide how to proceed.

The second half of the lessons we learned from Tim Ding, is listening. Listening is an art form many people require help in perfecting. Listening, being a part of a community, or volunteering takes time, effort, and an ability to listen to those around you.

When Tim Ding was confined to a bed in his home the women who were caring for him took the time to listen. They understood his resistance to their religious beliefs yet listening was a type of prayer for them. The respect they showed Tim was about him as a human, it was also a gentle lesson in how to participate in community. As you practice listening to others, you increase your compassion, empathy, and understanding. As a patient, family member, partner, or caregiver, when you slow down and actually hear what the other person is saying, without presuming, you give yourself and others the gift of clarity. With clarity comes ease. Even if you don't like what the other person is telling you, at least you are clear.

By removing the tendency to jump to conclusions, you greatly reduce the irritation, anger, resentment, and heartache that accompanies negative and confused emotions. Healing ceases in these common reactions. Who knew listening could boost your immune system?

I first learned of the term *Active Listening* while on retreat at Plumb Village in Bordeaux, France. Plumb Village is the home of Thích Nhất Hạnh, a Vietnamese Buddhist monk and peace activist. *Active Listening* is one of the many techniques used in Plumb Village to connect with others. It trains your brain to listen to the words people are saying. Often, we are listening simply to find the moment when WE can jump in to speak and express our opinion. To *actively listen* may sound counter-intuitive, but that couldn't be further from the truth. *Active Listening* takes considerably more effort than what we traditionally consider "listening."

Why You Should Try Active Listening:
Fighting for Your Marriage
by Howard J. Markman, Scott M. Stanley, Susan L Blumberg

Often, we'll listen to a partner without really hearing them.
In the process, we miss opportunities to connect with that person and even risk making them feel neglected, disrespected, and resentful. This exercise helps you express active interest in what the other person has to say and make them feel heard. It's a way to foster empathy and connection. This technique is especially well-suited for difficult conversations (such as arguments with a spouse) and for expressing support. Research suggests that using this technique can help others feel more understood and improve relationship satisfaction.

The Art of Active Listening
Time Required - 10 minutes per day for at least one week.
Find a quiet place where you can talk with a partner without interruption or distraction. Invite him or her to share what's on his or her mind. As he or she does so, try to follow the steps below. You don't need to cover every step, but the more you do cover, the more effective this practice is likely to be.

Paraphrase
Once the other person has finished expressing a thought, paraphrase/reflect what he or she said to make sure you understand and to show that you are paying attention. Helpful ways to paraphrase include, "What I hear you saying is..." "It sounds like..." and "if I understand you right...."

Closely repeating or paraphrasing what the speaker has said demonstrates comprehension, reinforcing the message they are trying to convey.

When our words are repeated by another, it helps solidify the message. Our words are powerful and often misunderstood by others. By repeating them to the speaker, they have the opportunity to hear them from the perspective of the receiver.

Ask questions

When appropriate, ask questions to encourage the other person to elaborate on his or her thoughts and feelings. It demonstrates that their listener has been paying attention by asking relevant questions and/or making statements that build or help to clarify what the speaker has said. Avoid jumping to conclusions about what the other person means. Instead, ask questions to clarify his or her meaning, such as, "When you say__, do you mean"? By asking relevant questions the listener also helps to reinforce that they have an interest in what the speaker has been saying.

Express empathy

If the other person voices negative feelings, strive to validate these feelings rather than questioning or defending against them. For example, if the speaker expresses frustration, try to consider why they feel that way, regardless of whether you think the feeling is justified or whether you would feel that way yourself were you in his or her position. You might respond, "I can sense that you're feeling frustrated," and even, "I can understand how that situation could cause frustration."

Use engaged body language

Show that you are engaged and interested by making eye contact, nodding, facing the other person, and maintaining an open and relaxed body posture. Avoid attending to distractions in your environment or checking your phone. Be mindful of your facial expressions. Avoid expressions that might communicate disapproval or disgust.

Avoid judgment

Your goal is to understand the other person's perspective and accept it for what it is, even if you disagree with it. Try not to interrupt with counter arguments or mentally preparing a rebuttal while the other person is speaking.

Avoid giving advice

Problem-solving is likely to be more effective after both partners understand one another's perspective and feel heard. Moving too quickly into advice-giving can be counterproductive.

Take turns

After the other person has had a chance to speak and you have engaged in the active listening steps above, ask if it's okay for you to share your perspective. When sharing your perspective, express yourself as clearly as possible using "I" statements (e.g., "I feel overwhelmed when you don't help out around the house"). It may also be helpful, when relevant, to express empathy for the other person's perspective (e.g., "I know you've been very busy lately and don't mean to leave me hanging...").

Evidence that it Works:

It's been documented in studies that participants who had brief conversations either with someone trained to engage in active listening, someone who gave them advice, or someone who gave simple acknowledgments of their point of view, reported feeling more understood at the end of the conversation.

Why it Works

Active listening helps listeners to better understand the other's perspective and helps (the) speaker feel more understood and less threatened. This technique can prevent miscommunication and spare hurt feelings on both sides. By improving communication and preventing arguments from escalating, active listening can make relationships more enduring and satisfying. Practicing active listening with someone close to you can also help you listen better when interacting with other people in your life.

I invite you to give active listening a try. It takes some practice and dedication to break the habit of interrupting or talking over others, but I assure you, it will make a difference in all your relationships. At first, you might even find people are confused by your ability to listen. It's an art that has been lost to our modern-day world.

Over the years, Tim Ding continues to volunteer his time, new communities and give back to others in new and expansive ways. His health, grace, and infectious laugh are as robust as ever.

Sources
Benefits of Volunteering:
https://www.helpguide.org/articles/healthy-living/volunteering-and-its-surprising-benefits.htm

Lissa Rankin Health Benefits of Finding Your Tribe:
http://lissarankin.com/the-health-benefits-of-finding-your-tribe

Active Listening:
ihttps://ggia.berkeley.edu/practice/active_listening
Instructions adapted from Markman, H., Stanley, S., & Blumberg, S.L. (1994).
Fighting for your marriage. San Francisco: Josey-Bass Publishers.

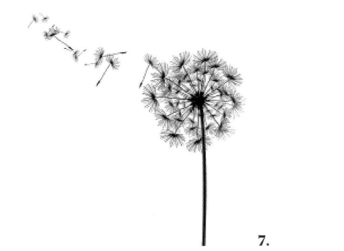

7.   Luisa

The Price of Perfectionism

I met Luisa on a beach in Barcelona Spain. We were seated across from one another for a Spanish-English language exchange event. I quickly discovered Luisa has a curiosity for all aspects of life. She's brilliant, affectionate, with a grace and wisdom that defy age. She possesses a unique ability to make you believe in yourself and the richness of life. Her smile and honesty radiate from within, because of this innate ease, I assumed her life had been easy and as joyful as she was. I was about to learn that people, even ones who are beautiful and quick-to-smile, are rarely one dimensional. Far from an uncomplicated life, I discovered how perfectionism, fear, and cancer actually transformed her life. Her lessons, inspire and offer hope for anyone experiencing the paralyzing anxiety that often accompanies a cancer journey.

Take a deep breath, smile and meet Luisa...

Luisa...

I woke in the middle of the night in excruciating pain. In the hours since I'd fallen asleep, I had developed a large lump on my neck. It was the first day of a new school year, and as a devoted teacher in Madrid, Spain, the work and students were my priority. I didn't have time to be sick.

I assumed the lump and pain would subside as quickly as it had developed. For the next few weeks my neck hurt, and depending on the day I felt exhausted, mildly tired, or a combination of both. Eventually, I went to the doctor; the results of a biopsy came back the day before the end of the first term.

Diagnosis: Hodgkin's Lymphoma.

The treatment protocol was aggressive. At the beginning I had fear, however, the doctor was hopeful, as this type of cancer responds well to chemo. Anxiety would subside and then reappear on days when I had to have an operation to insert a catheter or start a new treatment. Over time, fear lost its paralyzing grip on me, as if the fear had drifted quietly off to sleep. I knew it was there, however, I replaced it with thoughts of hope. I turned to courage and practiced being calm. I knew I had to be strong, fear was no longer useful to my healing. My belief in recovery was a priority. I was consciously changing how I reacted when I felt fearful, I learned to be in control. It wasn't easy, it came gradually, but I did eventually shift my belief about myself and my cancer.

It was important for me to continue working. I love teaching and I felt that if I was at work, I was normal. More than anything, I wanted to feel normal. I believed if my life remained as it was, having cancer would be easier to handle, or perhaps it was a way to deny cancer existed in my body. The doctor made a deal with me. He said; "Have your first chemo and after that, you can decide if you want to go back to work." It was evident after the first treatment: working would be impossible. I had to let go of the belief that teaching would make having cancer bearable.

Initially, it was difficult taking time off. I made a decision to look at recovery as my job. I had to figure out a way to come to terms with cancer. During this process, I was surprised to discover I was good without working. I realized for the first time, there was more to me than my work.

Shortly after my diagnosis, I had an interesting conversation with my doctor. He asked me if I was a perfectionist and self-demanding. When I said I was, he told me that Hodgkin's Lymphoma sometimes appears in people who have these qualities. I'd never considered my behaviour could have negative consequences on my health. I felt guilty and thought, even if I recover this could happen to me again. I needed to learn how to filter events, to relax, to be calm. Now I had time to consider my personality and belief systems.

For instance, I used to love to play the piano. I quit because I wasn't able to enjoy playing. The reason being was I needed to be perfect at it. I treated every lesson as an exam. I felt guilty if I hadn't practiced enough. It was a kind of punishment of myself, for not having the time to practice. My teacher couldn't understand me. If I was not prepared for the lesson or exam, then I believed I could never play perfectly. The teacher told me, "If you haven't practiced, that's ok with me, play the piano for the enjoyment of it." I said, "No, if I don't practice, I can't play, even for the pure pleasure of it."

I quit playing altogether. The joy of playing was swallowed by my perfectionism. Isn't that ridiculous!

Cancer and the lessons I learned about myself taught me how to live my life. The transition from an attitude of rigidity to one of acceptance has been the biggest adjustment for me. It didn't happen immediately – I had to examine myself and those around me. At one particularly low point, I spent five days crying. My mother always says, "Crying is not useful." but I believe it can be therapeutic, liberating and freeing, in moderation. I learned to be pragmatic, to focus on my priorities, to pay attention to myself. It was difficult because, in order to do this, I had to be selfish. I had to consider what is it I want. What was best for me and how to adjust my perfectionistic tendencies, use them for my benefit, instead of them using me.

I had to believe the changes I was making would be better for me, my friends, students, and parents, as a result of those changes, almost all of my relationships changed as a result. That felt overwhelmingly selfish. I had to find a way to not feel scared about being selfish. I needed to strike a balance between caring for myself and worrying about what my relationships would look like.

When your motivation is focused on others, it has little to do with being selfish, you do what you believe is best for them. This time, I had to change for me. I had to develop the unfamiliar belief that I deserved to change, which felt uncomfortable and extremely vulnerable. When you have cancer, you feel powerless; physically, emotionally and medically. Relying on others' opinions and advice is essential. Moving forward, I had to discover and decipher what I wanted and how I wanted to show up in the world.

Some of the relationships I had in my life were toxic. I had to decode which ones were healthy and step away from others. I needed to stay positive. I decided to surround myself with positivity, joy and a *lot of smiling.*

I was a serious child growing up, I was not really what anyone would consider happy. I recall one time when I was very little playing with my dolls, I had the thought, "Why am I in the world?" I was a bit of a philosopher at a young age and I remember thinking, "If I'm here then I have to do something good in the world." Perhaps that's why I became a teacher.

Cancer helped me discover I was stronger than I thought, and that I could hold that strength for others in my life, too. I felt that my mother was suffering a lot emotionally because of my illness. Somehow, this allowed me to let go of my fear and my need to be perfect. Cancer helped me realize that I could deal with anything. Cancer was the worst and the best thing I've been through in my life.

When the doctor told me, "The cancer is gone," I remember leaving the hospital and walking down the street with a huge smile on my face. I was looking at people smiling and feeling this power. It felt like I was superwoman because I felt like a hero...I was a survivor. A smiling, joyful survivor...

It's interesting, how my students always say to me now, "you're always happy" and of course, this isn't true. I explain to them, "I'm not always happy, I have good days and I have difficult ones. However, I like my life and I like my work, and this helps me to smile and feel happy." I tell them, "I know that if I come into class and don't smile, then you don't smile back at me and what's the point in life if you aren't connecting with others and spreading a little joy?" It's been my experience that if you believe you are happy, then you become happier.

The tiny things that come along don't bother me now. I can discriminate between what is worthy of my time, and worry and what isn't, but I still need to be vigilant and aware of stress. In my spare time, I love to study languages and challenge myself in new ways. I'm disciplined, and at times that discipline can lead to excessive pressure and I'm unable to relax. Then I feel tired. To me, being tired is a trigger related to cancer. That's when the fear returns. When I feel excessively tired, I tell myself, "It's not the cancer, you have to slow down, you are doing too many things, you have to relax. You can't study your languages, you can't go to the gym, you have to simply relax."

It's not easy to detect though. Once I realize I'm stressed it takes me a day or two to slow down and re-center myself.

I'm still a bit of a perfectionist and I like to be in control. However, I have learned that there are some things in life you can't control. I discovered life is a path with many choices, distractions, and decisions that are difficult to unravel. Perhaps these lessons come with age, but I had this experience with cancer, and I'll never know who I would have been without it. Remember what's important to you, consider other people, but make the final decision based on what is best for you.

Another thing I realized after cancer was that I began to naturally smile more and that change in me has been interesting because before cancer I was so serious, a little judgemental, and not overly sociable. What I learned about smiling is that it leads to gratitude. Being grateful helps me relax, and when I'm relaxed and calm, I can listen. Through listening, I'm a better person for myself and others.

Cancer has many demands, one of them is that you learn about yourself – but only if you *want* to learn.

If you don't want to learn, then you don't and that's a choice too.

For me, cancer taught me a multitude of lessons, most of all that I had choices to make that helped me evolve into the person I am today.

I chose to learn about myself.

I chose to grow through a daily dose of appreciation for myself and gratitude for others.

I chose to change habits that were too rigid.

By softening within myself, I discovered my OUTER and more importantly my *INNER SMILE*.

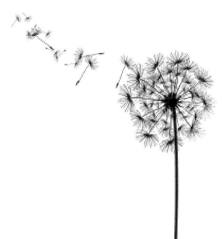

8. Using Fear to Motivate

Facing one's mortality at any age is a monumental task. Facing it in your twenties, as Luisa did, slams into you with an urgency to attain a lifetime of unrealized milestones, on a limited timeline that once appeared almost infinite.

The thought of never achieving one's purpose, finding the love of your life, having children or reaching your potential, is a staggering price to pay for illness.

It doesn't take long for patients to discover that cancer refuses to participate in bipartisan negotiations. Cancer is unwilling to discuss terms for good behaviour, time served, or genuine cooperation. The physical and emotional demands of cancer strike fear in the hearts of the tenacious and the tender alike. Fear is cancer's greatest ally. When you are under the smothering blanket of fear, it's the body's job to slow down your immune system to save energy in order to run or fight. A secondary job of fear is to impair your cognitive ability to reason or make rational decisions because these take effort and energy. In addition, your zest for living is doused, as survival becomes your body's primary task.

Cancer counts on this response; it uses fear to gain strength over your will, commanding unwavering respect and attention. Cancer uses fear like a toxic lover, swindling you into the belief that this is all your fault. It must be something you did or didn't do to cause all this dis-harmony. The length of time you stay wrapped in its all-consuming embrace is a choice only you can make. Options for eliminating fear are as diverse as the fear itself. Identifying the layers of fear, and addressing them one layer at a time, is generally considered to be easier, however, like that toxic love relationship, sometimes you need to break all ties before the fear destroys you. No endless talking about cancer, no time spent with negative friends or family, and definitely, no belief in the destructive lies that fear feeds you.

Similar to devices used to modulate treatments in your body, there are tools to administer an effective vaccine against fear. As with radiation, it's necessary to strike directly at the source, use a suitable dosage, space the therapy at appropriate intervals, then allow time for healing.

There are numerous books written on positivity, power of gratitude, laughter, grounding, music therapy, law of attraction, to name a few. The basis for these non-traditional therapies, directed to overall well-being, have threads woven among them. Interestingly, the men and women I interviewed for this book followed a similar protocol when managing their inner healing.

- ✓ Take time to consider when and where you feel contentment and ease.
- ✓ Become aware of the people, places, and circumstances in which happiness, joy, and strength are constant.
- ✓ Focus on good emotions until they become second nature.

✓ When experiencing extreme stress or fear, increase the dosage of positive feelings, minute by minute, hour by hour, as required.

✓ Allow a bad day to wash over you, free from guilt.

Don't be deceived by the simplicity of these mental practices. Fear has a way of embedding itself deep within the fibre of life. From a young age we are taught about fear: strangers, traffic, the boogeyman, disease, (in particular, cancer) and death. It requires constant vigilance to change these deeply rooted beliefs of the collective fear that cancer always equates to the end of life.

The fact is, illness has expressed itself in your body. But it is within your power to keep the malignancy called fear from invading your mind, too. Consider the strategies in this chapter to shift your focus away from illness and move it in the direction of ease. There will be strategies that resonate with you and others that don't. You are at choice. Isn't that lovely to hear for a change? You get to choose.

Below, when I refer to *the mind*, I'm not talking about your brain. The mind is in every cell, every thought, every moment, memory and experience you have or ever have had. Be it a conscious memory or an unconscious one. The mind is a set of cognitive faculties including perception, thought, judgment, memory, and consciousness. The mind holds the power of imagination, recognition, and appreciation. It is responsible for processing feelings and emotions, resulting in attitudes and actions. Is it any surprise the mind jumps to conclusions, sounding the alarm to fear all illness?

At the mere mention of cancer, the mental faculties of the mind stand at attention with acute cellular memory, all the information stored in our memory that isn't even necessarily true, yet, our collective mind can't process all the data, so it chooses to believe all of it. Every thought you've ever had about cancer comes to the forefront when a diagnosis is given.

When you are in a state of fear your ability to reason shuts down and instincts go on high alert. In this heightened state, the job of fear is to protect you. Fear defends you by telling you things that haven't happened are actual facts, such as; Cancer kills – Cancer always hurts – There is no cure – No one ever survives. Truth doesn't matter to fear because it is fear's job to protect you in a time of crisis by limiting your choices; choices such as running away, fighting back, or standing still. Also known as the Fight – Flight – Freeze response.

Fear has one job: to keep you safe from harm. What fear can't do is help you grasp that you have strength beyond any test results, beyond cold hard facts, beyond a frightening diagnosis. Fear raises your heart rate, spikes blood pressure, and slows digestion among other reactionary physical responses. Science has now proven beyond a doubt that humans have the ability to lower heart rate and blood pressure by thinking pleasant thoughts. When you do, your heart rate slows, fear subsides, and blood pressure returns to normal. In turn, your body returns to homeostasis, the state where your body works, your mind can reason, and the immune system heals illness.

I can only imagine, that at the time of diagnosis, you have zero access to pleasant thoughts. Ok, but let's assume you are past the stage of diagnosis. The shock has abated slightly, and decisions need to be made. Find a memory that used to make you smile. One significant or fleeting situation, person or event which, when you ease into it, your body responds by calming down.

It could be the memory of a spectacular sunset, the smile of a loved one, compassion from a stranger, anything that produces a feeling of joy. There's this delicious involuntary reaction when you recall a pleasant thought. It inhabits your consciousness, the cells that were mobilized to help you experience the event when it happened are re-activated, just by thinking about it. The body believes that it's happening in the here and now. It's a bit of a mind-hack that you can use for your enjoyment, or on the flip-side, when your thoughts land on an anxious or troubling event, and those fearful memory cells are ignited, heart-rate quickens, your blood pressure rises, digestion slows and fear is remembered in your mind and in your entire body.

In simple terms, you go into fight-flight-freeze and all healing ceases.

This is your mind doing some of its best work. Our thoughts have the ability to physically expand the experience from a mere thought, to the belief that it's happening in the present moment. Of course, you know intellectually that it's not going on now, but your body responds to emotionally charged memories with exacting accuracy. With pleasant memories, you are bathed in the experience of joy, happiness, gratitude, love, etc. Your body naturally moves into the cellular memory of being at-ease. The exact mirroring effect occurs when fearful memories are triggered, is activated. Use this mind-hack to combat fear when it threatens your very existence by altering the impact your body and cells must endure.

By returning to a pleasant thought, experience or memory, you allow your mind to access those endorphins that reside in states of joy, happiness, love, gratitude, kindness, or any emotion that feels good to you. Those feelings activate your healing. The body wants more of those good feelings, and in order to provide it, your cells need to be in a loving rejuvenative state so you can access the natural condition of health.

Have you ever noticed that when you are experiencing fearful thoughts that you spiral into a swamp of negativity, triggering a cascade of negative thoughts, often without a single basis in truth? When pessimistic and fearful thoughts take hold of your intellectual reasoning, it signals the amygdala *(a primal section of the brain responsible for detecting fear and preparing for emergency events, such as combat with and enemy tribe or fending off an approaching threat)*. The amygdala jumps into action in order to protect you from a threatening event, be it real or imagined. The purpose of the amygdala in any stressful situation is to suppress your metabolism and immune system, allowing adrenaline to flood your cells.

This action initiates your inner protection system. Fear – of any kind – triggers the adrenal gland to pump cortisol into the bloodstream. This is known as the sympathetic nervous system, which removes your ability to achieve peace and tranquility, the very mindset where healing takes place. Family members and friends experience a similar response to a loved one facing illness, often, they are too involved to notice their overall wellbeing is threatened too.

The amygdala – unevolved since caveman days – is primal in its reaction, it hasn't evolved past caveman days, unable to decipher or prioritize threats. It's unlikely the majority of us will ever have to fight neighbouring tribesmen or flee from an advancing saber-toothed tiger, yet a cancer patient is living with their own version of an enemy-tribe, and saber-toothed tiger, on a regular basis.

Initiating strategies to overcome fear will assist you in healing. The good news; THE CHOICE IS YOURS. This is not about your partner, parents, siblings, best friends or caregivers. This is a time when it's all about YOU. Yes, you must consider your loved ones, but this is your body and your recovery. You've had to make many decisions since your diagnosis and many of you have had decisions forced upon you. That's the nature of living with cancer. It wasn't your choice.

Here and now relax for a moment, take a slow deep breath, and turn your attention on you. Not on your illness, not on your life, on. Take some time to think about what brings you joy and happiness. Sit with it and recall the details. Where were you, what was the time of year, were you in a room, outside, on holiday? Replay it like a movie in your head. Remember it in as much detail as possible.

I've listed several suggestions below. Pick one or two of the suggestions below that resonate with you. And be kind to yourself. If you struggle with any of these techniques or if one or more of them don't feel good to you, simply choose another. Take breaks. Try again tomorrow or next week. Removing criticism and judgment from your daily thought patterns assists you in your healing. Do what works for you.

Recover some of the power you surrendered to this disease. Through loving acts of kindness to yourself, you'll regain or find for the first time, inner strength.

FEAR REDUCING STRATEGIES:

Meditation:
Meditating can occur in many forms. Walking in nature,

riding a bicycle, drinking the perfect cup of coffee or by calming the mind and body on a meditation pillow. A large body of research on one particular type of meditation called Metta, also referred to as Loving Kindness Meditation. An extensive study of Buddhist monks in Metta Meditation have proven scientifically to rewire the brain and quiet the amygdala. And it doesn't take much time or experience.

If you've never meditated before, expect it will take a little practice. Be kind to yourself, don't expect to channel Buddha in the first week. Meditation is similar to a muscle. It must be strengthened in order for it to flourish and become a practice. The good news is, small increments have the ability to produce massive results.

How long you actually need to meditate is a bit subjective. Start with one minute, move to five minutes. The average meditation lasts between 5-25 minutes. I've personally practiced for a little as 10 seconds. Even that snippet of time eases my stress and calms me in difficult or fearful situations. It's not the time, location or type of meditation you practice. It's in the doing. A little like standing next to the pool and thinking about swimming, you'll never learn to swim until you get yourself in the water.

Like being in the pool, it's not important what you do once you're bobbing around; the fact you made it there in the first place is worth celebrating. As you spend more time in meditation, you'll come to a place of comfort and ease. You'll find what works best for you. Every second you spend in meditation brings you closer to aligning with optimum physical, mental and emotional wellbeing. The beauty of healing through meditation is that it's simple.

If at any time it becomes work...stop and try again the next hour or the following day. Ease into it gently. Be kind to yourself. It's been said that the magic of meditation is between the gap.

The gap between your heartbeat...
The gap between thinking...
The gap between doing...

HERE'S A QUICK START GUIDE TO METTA MEDITATION:

Find a comfortable chair, pillow, folded blanket or prepare a dedicated meditation nest in your home.

If you like, light a candle or some incense. Feel free to surround yourself with a few favourite objects, such as seashells, rocks, cards or mementos of any kind, that calm you.

I have a spot on my sofa – I drape a cozy blanket over my knees and in the winter a heated bean bag sits in my lap. Prior to meditating, I prepare a cup of ginger tea as a little reward

Take time to consider what gives you comfort, allows you to relax. The meditating becomes a joy instead of another thing on your To-Do List.

Sit in a cross-legged meditation position, on a chair, laying down or any place that's comfortable for you. (I personally don't lay down, as meditation puts me to sleep.

Keep your back straight. Eyes can be closed or softly focused on an object such as a plant or the flickering flame of a candle.

Take two deep breaths, followed by your normal breathing pattern.

Take a moment to notice the feeling of the rise and fall of your chest or abdomen.

Feel the cushion or chair beneath you.

Imagine yourself connected to the earth with roots growing beneath you, that hold you sturdy and safe.

Begin by developing loving-kindness towards yourself. This isn't a traditional mantra, it is not to be repeated mechanically, but mindfully, with full awareness, knowing what you're saying, feeling the intention behind the good wishes; the feeling and intention behind each phrase.

Repeat the following affirmations three times:

1. - May I be Safe
   - May I be Peaceful and Happy
   - May I be Healthy
   - May I Live with Ease & Grace

2. - May I be Safe
   - May I be Peaceful and Happy
   - May I be Healthy
   - May I Live with Ease & Grace

3. - May I be Safe
   - May I be Peaceful and Happy
   - May I be Healthy
   - May I Live with Ease & Grace

Next: Choose a loved one and say these words to yourself 3 times:
  - May you be Safe
  - May you be Peaceful and Happy
  - May you be Healthy
  - May you Live with Ease & Grace – Repeat 3 Times

Next: Think of a friend.

Bring their face to mind, imagine them smiling and receiving your wishes:
  - May you be Safe
  - May you be Peaceful and Happy
  - May you be Healthy
  - May you Live with Ease & Grace – Repeat 3 Times

Next: Think of a neutral person who you have limited contact with or know only casually. I rotate between a homeless man who lives in my neighbourhood, to someone who I've come in contact with, but don't actually know their name.
  - May you be Safe
  - May you be Peaceful and Happy
  - May you be Healthy
  - May you Live with Ease & Grace – Repeat 3 Times

The next one has the potential to trigger your emotions, so go slowly and easily at first.

Choose a person in your life who's hurt you, a person you've never come to a resolution about it.

You know if you have the right person or event when you remember it like it was yesterday. But as a caution here, if this becomes painful, pick someone else, ease into those difficult people, topics, and situations – gradually.

This is not an exercise in making what they did ok or even forgiving them...what you are attempting to do is find a place deep inside where you can wish them the common decency to which all humans are entitled to, even beyond the unforgivable.

This exercise is for you, not them, keep that in mind. No need to revisit the offence. Eventually, the pain and suffering that happened in the past will be discharged. Getting stuck in these destructive repetitive patterns causes you additional anguish and suffering and it slows healing.

Think of the person who hurt you and begin by saying:
- May you be Safe
- May you be Peaceful and Happy
- May you be Healthy
- May you Live with Ease & Grace – Repeat 3 Times

Lastly, imagine all sentient beings. Anyone or anything who can think or feel.
- May you be Safe
- May you be Peaceful and Happy
- May you be Healthy
- May you Live with Ease & Grace – Repeat 3 Time

Metta Meditation is quick, easy and effective! Try it for a few weeks. If you really don't like it, stop, try something different. This is not about forcing yourself. But be open to finding a quiet place within, breathe in the beauty of life and soothe your soul in the process. Your body does its best healing when you are in a place of peace. Focus on a desire for happiness and wellbeing for all. Recite specific words or sentences that evoke boundless warm-hearted feeling of happiness and peace.

To recap the stages of Metta

1. Self – *3 repetitions of May I Be Safe – May I Be Peaceful and Healthy – May I Live with Ease and Grace*

2. **Loved One** – *(family member, partner, cherished pet)* – *3 repetitions of May You Be Safe – May You Be Peaceful and Happy – May You be Healthy – May You Live with Ease and Grace*

3. **Friend** – *3 repetitions of May You Be Safe – May You Be Peaceful and Happy – May You be Healthy – May You Live with Ease and Grace*

4. **"Neutral" person** (someone you have limited contact with, or know only casually) – *3 repetitions of May You Be Safe – May You Be Peaceful and Happy – May You be Healthy – May You Live with Ease and Grace*

5. **A Difficult person from your past, or someone you are currently having a challenge with.** – *3 repetitions of May You Be Safe – May You Be Peaceful and Happy – May You be Healthy – May You Live with Ease and Grace*

6. **The Entire Universe** – *3 repetitions of May You Be Safe – May You Be Peaceful and Happy – May You be Healthy – May You Live with Ease and Grace*

If this feels too cumbersome, Guided Meditations are another good place to start. My personal favourites are Jon Kabat- Zinn, Davidji, or Thich Nhat Hanh, they all can be found on YouTube. Find someone whose voice you like and trust. Be sure that you enjoy the flow and rhythm of their voice, and their music if they use it. You'll find free recordings on YouTube, Soundcloud,

Headspace and your local Library. You could ask a friend to recommend a CD, mp3 or video.

For some meditators, watching beautiful landscapes online helps them or focusing on an object, like a candle, stills the mind. I prefer closing my eyes, but it's up to you. Play with what works. Even one minute of clearing the mind chatter will positively boost your overall well-being.

The best and brightest meditation teachers agree that HOW is not important, it's the experience of calm and tranquility that you are striving for. Whether it lasts a 1 minute or an hour isn't the point.

All meditation is significant
With practice, you will find the balance that works best for you. There are as many kinds of meditations as there are ways to practice: BodyMind, Visual, Zen, Sound, Energy, Sensory, Buddhist, Mantra, Chanting, Walking, the list of ways to meditate is infinite. Pick one that resonates with you, see if it's a fit. If not try another.

One of the side-effects of meditation is it reduces pain. A research group from the *University of Montreal* exposed 13 Zen masters and 13 comparable non-practitioners to equal degrees of painful heat while measuring their brain activity in a functional magnetic resonance imaging (fMRI) scanner. What they discovered is that the Zen meditation (called zazen) practitioners reported less pain. Actually, they reported even less pain than their neurological output from the fMRI indicated. So even though their brain may be receiving the same amount of pain input, in their minds there is less pain. (Time Magazine, NCBI, David Lynch Foundation)

Meditation vs morphine

In an experiment conducted by Wake Forest Baptist Medical Centre, 15 healthy volunteers, who were new to meditation, attended four 20-minute classes to learn meditation, focusing on the breath. Both before and after meditation training, study participants' brain activity was examined using ASL MRI, while the pain was inflicted on them by using heat.

Fadel Zeidan, Ph.D., lead author of the study, explains that "This is the first study to show that only a little over an hour of meditation training can dramatically reduce both the experience of pain and pain-related brain activation. We found a big effect – about a 40 percent reduction in pain intensity and a 57 percent reduction in pain unpleasantness. **Meditation produced a greater reduction in pain than even morphine or other pain-relieving drugs, which typically reduce pain ratings by about 25 percent."**

2. Expressive Writing

Releasing one's feelings through writing or journaling (letters or diaries) is an ancient tradition, one that dates back to around 10th century Japan. Throughout history, civilization has used the written word to process inner conflict. It's been prescribed as a therapy for those suffering from depression, anger, anguish, fear, and trauma to name just a few. I love to write my feelings down through Expressive Writing when I'm in extreme distress, confusion or simply processing personal emotions.

In the book: *"Writing to Heal: A Guided Journal for Recovering from Trauma and Emotional Upheaval"*, Dr. James Pennebaker describes what he calls:

The Expressive Writing Method
   ✓ Find a time and place where you won't be disturbed.

✓ Promise yourself you will write continuously for at least 15-20 minutes each day, for 3-4 consecutive days.

✓ Don't worry about spelling or grammar.

✓ If you run out of things to say, repeat what you just wrote.

✓ Write only for yourself. Confidentiality is key to uncensored writing. (when privacy is an issue, burning or shredding your pages are advised)

✓ Write about something extremely personal and important for you.

✓ Deal only with events or situations you can handle now.

✓ You can write longhand or type on a computer. If you are unable to write, speak into a recording device.

✓ You can write about the same thing each day or something different each day. It's entirely up to you.

What to Write About:

✓ Something that you are thinking or worrying about too much.

✓ Something that you are dreaming about.

✓ Something that you feel is affecting your life in an unhealthy way.

✓ Something that you have been avoiding for days, weeks, or years.

As a cautionary note, Pennebaker suggests not attempting to write about trauma too soon after it happens. *"If a topic seems like it's too much to handle, don't try to tackle it before you're ready. The effects of writing can be subtle, but sometimes they can be dramatic."*

Through his extensive research, Dr. Pennebaker generally gives people the following instructions for writing:

"Over the next four days, I want you to write about your deepest emotions and thoughts about the most upsetting experience in your life. Really let go and explore your feelings and thoughts about it. In your writing, you might tie this experience to your childhood, your relationship with your parents, people you have loved or love now, your career or your illness. How is this experience related to who you would like to become, who you have been in the past, or who you are now?"

"Some people have not had a single traumatic experience, others have had many, but all of us have had major conflicts or stressors in our lives and you can write about them as well. You can write about the same issue every day or a series of different issues. Whatever you choose to write about, it is critical that you really let go and explore your very deepest emotions and thoughts."

Warning: *"Many people report that after writing, they sometimes feel somewhat sad or depressed. Like seeing a sad movie, this typically goes away in a couple of hours. If you find that you are getting extremely upset about a writing topic, simply stop writing or change topics."*

Dr. Pennebaker's extensive studies have shown:

"When people are given the opportunity to write about emotional upheavals, they often experience improved health. They go to the doctor less and have an improvement in immune function."

3. Emotional Freedom Technique - EFT

EFT is also referred to as Tapping, it draws many of its principles from the ancient healing lineage of Traditional Chinese medicine. (*I'll refer to it as Tapping for simplicity sake*)

So far, modern science's investigations into just why **Tapping works have been astounding.**

The results revealed why Tapping is the perfect bridge between cutting edge Western medicine and ancient healing practices from the East. For example, studies at Harvard Medical School have revealed that by stimulating the body's meridian points – the same spots on your body that are manipulated by acupuncturists – you can significantly reduce activity in a part of your brain called the amygdala. Think of your amygdala as a personal alarm system.

When you experience trauma or fear, the amygdala is triggered and your body is flooded with cortisol, commonly known as the "stress hormone." This intricate chain reaction – your stress response – significantly influences, and sometimes even causes, whatever it is that troubles you: whether that's an illness, a relationship, an injury, or even an external problem such as your finances. These studies show that by stimulating these parts of your body – as we do in Tapping – you can drastically reduce or eliminate the distress that accompanies or gives rise to these problems you face. By so doing, you can often eliminate the problems themselves! Below I give you an explanation of What tapping is from the homepage of Nick Ortner's website The Tapping Solution.

He explains it in detail and better than I ever could. For additional information, go to their website or better yet watch their YouTube video, type in: *Tapping 101 – Learn the Basics of the Tapping Technique.*
https://thetappingsolution.com/tapping-101

What is tapping?
(The Tapping Solution homepage)
Millions of people are settling for lives filled with poor health and emotional baggage. Not knowing how to achieve the joyful and satisfying lives they desire, they're stuck accepting a lifestyle of

emotional trauma, chronic physical pain, compulsions, and addictions, or perhaps just an empty feeling inside. Along with these problems come pills to kill the pain, sleep at night, and suppress anxiety – but this is hardly better than the disease.

If you're like many people, you feel trapped, caught in this cycle. You're tired of feeling sad, depressed, anxious, discontent, and unwell. You're sick of expensive and ineffective treatments. You're fed up with relinquishing the power over your health and happiness to psychologists and doctors. You'd like to grow, flourish, and thrive, putting the past in the past. You want to be your best, living a life that is filled with peace, joy, and fulfillment, from day to day and moment to moment.

With Tapping, you can do that. You can discover the vital secret for emotional wholeness and physical relief. You can take your physical and emotional well-being into your own hands. It's simple for anyone to master, and it's free.

Tapping provides relief from chronic pain, emotional problems, disorders, addictions, phobias, post-traumatic stress disorder, and physical diseases. While Tapping is newly set to revolutionize the field of health and wellness, the healing concepts that it's based upon have been in practice in Eastern medicine for over 5,000 years. Like acupuncture and acupressure, Tapping is a set of techniques which utilize the body's energy meridian points. You can stimulate these meridian points by tapping on them with your fingertips – literally tapping into your body's own energy and healing power.

Your body is more powerful than you can imagine...filled with life, energy, and a compelling ability for self-healing. With Tapping, you can take control of that power.

So How Does It All Work?

All negative emotions are felt through a disruption of the body's energy. And physical pain and disease are intricately connected to negative emotions. Health problems create feedback – physical symptoms cause emotional distress, and unresolved emotional problems manifest themselves through physical symptoms. So, the body's health must be approached as a whole. You cannot treat the symptoms without addressing the cause, and vice-versa.

The body, like everything in the universe, is composed of energy. Restore balance to the body's energy, and you will mend the negative emotions and physical symptoms that stem from the energy disruption. Tapping restores the body's energy balance, and negative emotions are conquered.

The basic technique requires you to focus on the negative emotion at hand: a fear or anxiety, a bad memory, an unresolved problem, or anything that's bothering you. While maintaining your mental focus on this issue, use your fingertips to tap 5-7 times each on 12 of the body's meridian points. Tapping on these meridian points – while concentrating accepting and resolving the negative emotion – will access your body's energy, restoring it to a balanced state.

You may be wondering about these meridians. Put simply, energy circulates through your body along a specific network of channels. You can tap into this energy at any point along the system.

This concept comes from the doctrines of traditional Chinese medicine, which referred to the body's energy as "ch'i." In ancient times, the Chinese discovered 100 meridian points. They also discovered that by stimulating these meridian points, they could heal. Call it energy, call it the Source, call it life force, call it ch'i...Whatever you want to call it, it works.

In some ways, Tapping is similar to acupuncture. Like Tapping, acupuncture achieves healing through stimulating the body's meridians and energy flow. However, unlike Tapping, acupuncture involves needles! "No needles" is definitely one of the advantages of Tapping.

Acupuncture also takes years to master. Acupuncture practitioners must memorize hundreds of meridian points along the body; the knowledge and training take years to acquire.

Tapping is simple and painless. It can be learned by anyone. And you can apply it to yourself, whenever you want, wherever you are. It's less expensive and less time-consuming. It can be used with specific emotional intent towards your own unique life challenges and experiences. Most importantly, it gives you the power to heal yourself, putting control over your destiny back into your own hands.

The Science Behind Tapping's Success

Like many healing arts that draw upon ancient wisdom, Tapping has been met with a fair share of skepticism. Many doctors and psychologists have been quick to dismiss it as "woo woo", despite the heaping anecdotal evidence from practitioners and people who have used EFT on their own.

In recent years, however, there's been a growing pool of undeniable research that proves what millions of people the world over have known for some time now: that EFT produces real, lasting breakthroughs and significantly improves or even eliminates conditions that hospital treatments, medication and years of psychotherapy often fail to adequately deal with.

Studies conducted at no less than Harvard Medical School verify these assertions. Research done at the prestigious university during the last decade found that the brain's stress and fear response – which is controlled by an almond-shaped part of your brain called the amygdala – could be lessened by stimulating the meridian points used in acupuncture, acupressure, and of course, tapping.

Although these studies focused on acupuncture and as such used needles, follow-up double-blind research revealed that stimulating the points through pressure, as we do in tapping, gave rise to a similar response!

Another exciting set of research was undertaken by Dr. Dawson Church. His team performed a randomized controlled trial to study how an hour-long tapping session would impact the stress levels of 83 subjects. To do this, Dr. Church and his team measured their level of cortisol, a hormone secreted by the body when it undergoes stress. Their findings? The average level of cortisol reduction was 24%, with a whopping reduction of almost 50% in some subjects! In comparison, there was no significant cortisol reduction in those who underwent an hour of traditional talk therapy.

Dr. Church also created *The Stress Project*, which teaches tapping to war veterans suffering from PTSD. The results have been astounding: an average 63% decrease in PTSD symptoms after six rounds of tapping. It's mind-blowing and exciting research, which has converted many non-believers in the scientific community along the way. All signs indicate that this trend of revealing research and swayed skeptics will continue as millions of people around the globe continue to discover the power of tapping.

The History of Tapping: An Accidental Discovery Leads to a Healing Revolution

It began in 1980, with a psychologist by the name of Roger Callahan, and a patient with an extreme phobia of water. Mary's fear of water controlled her life and kept her from daily activities. She was unable to take her children to the beach and was unable to drive near the ocean; she grew fearful when it rained and could not even withstand the sight of water on TV. She had vivid nightmares involving water.

Dr. Callahan and Mary had been working on this problem together for over a year. Finally, Mary worked up the courage to sit within sight of the pool at Dr. Callahan's house. Even doing this caused Mary extreme distress, and though she found ways to cope with the intense fear and emotional pain, she did not overcome her phobia. They discussed her problem, and how to overcome it, but without success.

Her fear of being near the water caused Mary stomach pains – a common "gut reaction." Dr. Callahan had recently been studying traditional Chinese medicines and learning about meridians. Suddenly he had an inspiration. Remembering that there was an acupuncture point for the stomach meridian on the cheekbone, he asked her to tap there, thinking it might cure her stomach pains.

Mary tapped her cheekbone as directed, and this little action changed medicinal history! The response seemed miraculous, to both Mary and Dr. Callahan. Her stomach pains disappeared. But even more amazingly, her phobia of water disappeared, too! She ran down to the pool and began splashing herself with water, rejoicing in her newfound freedom from fear.

Based on this discovery, Dr. Callahan began a series of investigations to develop and refine this technique, which he termed Thought Field Therapy. Gary Craig trained under Dr. Callahan's tutelage in the 1990s, learning the procedures for TFT. As time passed, Craig began to observe some problems with TFT, aspects that he saw were unnecessary complications. TFT required practitioners to tap on a specific sequence of meridians (called and algorithm) for each different problem.

Diagnosing the problem required a technique called muscle testing, wherein the practitioner would measure the relative strength of a muscle, while the patient explored various thoughts or statements.

Craig observed repeated scenarios in which the problem was incorrectly diagnosed, or the practitioner tapped out the meridian points in the wrong order, yet the patient was still helped. Based on these observations, he concluded that it did not matter in which order the meridian points were tapped.

Craig developed EFT as a simplified, improved version of the concepts behind Callahan's TFT. EFT has one basic, simple sequence of points to tap, no matter what the situation.

Because of this, thousands of people have used Tapping for illnesses and to resolve emotional problems. Tapping practitioners have studied the techniques and trained to take on more complicated and difficult cases, and these dedicated practitioners report more successful applications daily. More and more people are discovering and exploring Tapping. Many are discovering how Tapping can change their lives.

Basic Tapping Sequence for Anxiety

As discussed, Tapping can be used for everything – try it on everything! In this example, we'll focus on general anxiety. Try it now with this initial sequence.

Here's how a basic Tapping sequence works:

Identify the problem you want to focus on. It can be general anxiety, or it can be a specific situation or issue which causes you to feel anxious.

Consider the problem or situation. How do you feel about it right now? Rate the intensity level of your anxiety, with zero being the lowest level of anxiety and ten being the highest.

Compose your set up statement. Your set up statement should acknowledge the problem you want to deal with, then follow it with an unconditional affirmation of yourself as a person. (change the words below to suit your challenge at the moment)

"Even though I feel this anxiety, I deeply and completely accept myself."

"Even though I'm anxious about my interview, I deeply and completely accept myself."

"Even though I'm feeling this anxiety about my financial situation, I deeply and completely accept myself."

"Even though I panic when I think about, I deeply and completely accept myself."

"Even though I'm worried about how to approach my boss, I deeply and completely accept myself."

"Even though I'm having trouble breathing, I deeply and completely accept myself."

Perform the Setup

With four fingers on one hand, tap the Karate Chop point on your other hand. The Karate Chop point is on the outer edge of the hand, on the opposite side from the thumb.

Repeat the setup statement three times aloud, while simultaneously tapping the Karate Chop point. Now take a deep breath.

Get ready to begin tapping!

Here are some tips to help you achieve the right technique:

You should use a firm but gentle pressure as if you were drumming on the side of your desk or testing a melon for ripeness.

You can use all four fingers, or just the first two (the index and middle fingers). Four fingers are generally used on the top of the head, the collarbone, under the arm...wider areas. On sensitive areas, like around the eyes, you can use just two.

Tap with your fingertips, not your fingernails. The sound will be round and mellow.

The tapping order begins at the top and works down. You can end by returning to the top of the head, to complete the loop.

Now, tap 5-7 times each on the remaining eight points in the following sequence:

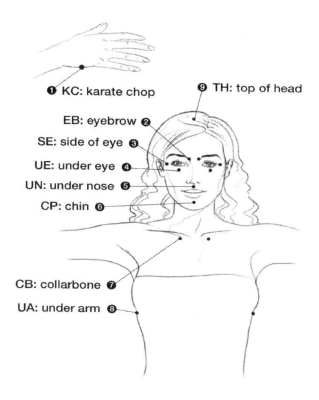

(image: www.thetappingsolution.com)

Head (TH)

The crown, centre and top of the head. Tap with all four fingers on both hands.

Eyebrow (EB)

The inner edges of the eyebrows, closest to the bridge of the nose. Use two fingers.

Side of eye (SE)

The hard area between the eye and the temple. Use two fingers. Feel out this area gently so you don't poke yourself in the eye!

Under-eye (UE)

The hard area under the eye, that merges with the cheekbone. Use two fingers, in line beneath the pupil.

Under nose (UN)

The point centered between the bottom of the nose and the upper lip. Use two fingers.

Chin (CP)

This point is right beneath the previous one and is centered between the bottom of the lower lip and the chin.

Collarbone (CB)

Tap just below the hard ridge of your collarbone with four fingers.

Underarm (UA)

On your side, about four inches beneath the armpit. Use four fingers.

Head (TH)

And back where you started, to complete the sequence.

As you tap on each point, repeat a simple reminder phrase, such as "my anxiety" or "my illness" or "my financial situation."

Now take another deep breath!

Now that you've completed the sequence, focus on your problem again. How intense is the anxiety now, in comparison to a few minutes ago? Give it a rating on the same number scale.

If your anxiety is still higher than "2", you can do another round of tapping. Keep tapping until the anxiety is gone. You can change your set up statement to take into account your efforts to fix the problem, and your desire for continued progress.

"Even though I have some remaining anxiety, I deeply and completely accept myself."

"Even though I'm still a little worried about this interview, I deeply and completely accept myself."
And so on.

Now that you've focused on dispelling your immediate anxiety, you can work on installing some positive feelings instead.

Note: This approach is different from traditional "positive thinking." You're not being dishonest with yourself. You're not trying to obscure the stress and anxiety inside yourself with a veneer of insincere affirmations. Rather, you've confronted and dealt with the anxiety and negative feelings, offering deep and complete acceptance to both your feelings and yourself. Now, you're turning your thoughts and vibrations to the powerful and positive.

That's what makes Tapping so much more effective than the "positive thinking" techniques that many of you have already tried. It's not just a mental trick; instead, you're using these positive phrases and tapping to tune into the very real energy of positivity, affirmation, and joy that is implicit inside you. You're actually changing your body's energy into a more positive flow, a more positive vibration.

Here are some example phrases to guide you:

"I have faith in my ability to change."

"I am joyful about these positive changes."
"I am accomplishing so much."
"I enjoy the calm and peace that I have."
"I love the person that I am."
"I am becoming a more relaxed and joyful person."

You can use these positive phrases with the same tapping points and sequences described above.

Congratulations! You've completed your first Tapping sequence.

Have Some Fun While Reducing Cortisol Levels
(From Lissa Rankin's bestselling book, *Mind Over Medicine*)

Laugh more:
In his bestselling book, *The Anatomy of An Illness*, Norman Cousins tells the story of how he cured himself from the debilitating condition ankylosing spondylitis by laughing along with Marx Brothers movies. He wrote, "I made the joyous discovery that ten minutes of genuine belly laughter had an anesthetic effect and would give me at least two hours of pain-free sleep. When the pain-killing effect of the laughter wore off, we would switch on the motion picture projector again and not infrequently, it would lead to another pain-free interval."

Play with animals:
Snuggling with our pets fills us with oxytocin, endorphins, and other healing hormones that support the body's self-healing mechanisms. This is why pet therapy can be so effective, both mentally and physically. So, go cuddle Fido or rub Fifi's belly, and

let them cut your cortisol levels while ramping up your body's capacity to self-repair.

Give generously:

When Cami Walker was diagnosed with debilitating multiple sclerosis, conventional medicine had very little to offer. Then a South African medicine woman suggested that instead of focusing on herself, she needed to shift towards thinking more about others. The medicine woman wrote Cami a prescription – Give 29 gifts in 29 days. So, she did. And as if by magic, her MS symptoms started to diminish. How? Because giving activates relaxation responses, which bolster the body's natural self-repair mechanisms.

Andy Mackey enjoyed similar health benefits from giving generously. After 9 heart surgeries, Andy's doctors had him on 15 medications, but the side effects made him miserable. So, he decided to stop all his medications and spend his remaining days feeling as good as he could. His doctors said he would die within a year, so Andy decided to do something he had always wanted to do. He decided to use the money he would have spent on his heart medicines to buy 300 harmonicas for children, with lessons. And when he didn't die the next month, he bought a few hundred more. It's now 11 years and 16,000 harmonicas later and Andy Mackey is still giving generously.

Express yourself creatively:

Creative expression releases endorphins and other feel-good neurotransmitters reduce depression and anxiety, improves your immune function, relieves physical pain, and activates the parasympathetic nervous system: thereby lowering your heart rate, decreasing your blood pressure, slowing down your breathing, and lowering cortisol.

Practice yoga, tai chi, Qigong, or dance forms like Gabrielle Roth's 5 Rhythms – or get a massage:

All of these modalities, which combine the benefits of exercise and meditation, steep you in healing hormones and have been proven to effectively drop cortisol levels and improve our body's ability to heal itself.

Or, get a massage – the ultimate relaxation response activator. A nurturing massage not only relaxes your muscles, but it also relaxes your nervous system and kicks those self-healing mechanisms into high gear.

Get it on:

Those with healthy sex lives live longer, have a lower risk of heart disease and stroke, get less breast cancer, enjoy the benefits fits of stronger immune systems, sleep better, appear more youthful, enjoy improved fitness, have enhanced fertility, get relief from chronic pain, experience fewer migraines, suffer from less depression, and enjoy an improved quality of life. Oh - and their cortisol levels are lower!

Pray or attend services as part of a spiritual community:

Those who attend religious services live up to 14 years longer than those who don't but don't go to church if it's not in alignment with your authentic beliefs. Find – or create – your own spiritual tribe and enjoy the hormonal benefits of gathering together with the intention of loving, healing, and lifting the vibration of each other and the planet. Your nervous system – and your body – will thank you.

Alleviate your loneliness:

Lonely people have twice the rate of heart disease as people who aren't lonely. In fact, loneliness researchers suggest that alleviating your loneliness is more important to a healthy life-style than quitting smoking or starting to exercise. As Robert Putnam put it in *Bowling Alone*, "As a rough rule of thumb, if you belong to no groups but decide to join one, you cut your risk of dying over the next year in half. If you smoke and belong to no groups, it's a toss-up statistically whether you should stop smoking or start joining. These findings are in some way heartening. It's easier to join a group than to lose weight, exercise regularly, or quit smoking."

Be brave enough to take radical action in order to reduce your stress responses:

Ask yourself, "What does my body need in order to heal?" If your intuition says, "You have to quit that soul-sucking job," or "You've got to get out of that abusive relationship," listen up. You've just written The Prescription for yourself. To learn more about how to write The Prescription for yourself, read Mind Over Medicine.

Too scared to take a leap of faith? Lissa and her colleagues suggest:

"If you want big miracles, you have to take big risks. If you're wanting to take smaller risks, you'll have to accept smaller miracles."

Grounding – Earthing

I absolutely love the idea behind Grounding also known as Earthing. When I was walking 800 km along The Camino de Santiago Trail, I naturally grounded myself several times a day. Whenever I stopped to rest, I'd remove my shoes and socks and touch the earth with my feet. I didn't know why I was doing it, I just felt better when my bare feet were touching the earth. It gave me energy and calmed me down. Unlike most people on The Camino, I never had problems with my knees, or my feet and I believe my quiet moments grounding my feet to the powerful earth had a lot to do with my lack of pain or discomfort. Not to mention, I was happy, joyful and grateful.

It was a little like while I was in Italy and sitting on the bench in the garden at Federica's. I was allowing the earth to transfer its gentle electric charge to me through my bare feet. Grounding is one of the quickest ways to feel better in the moment and to help your body and mind heal. Ever wonder why when you are on a beach holiday, you just feel better? It turns out it's because when you are on a beach holiday, you are often barefoot. No rubber soled shoes, asphalt, or buildings to break the current you and the healing benefits of mother nature.

I came across the book by Clint Ober entitled *Earthing - The Most Important Health Discovery Ever?* He's the man who brought Earthing to popular culture. Many have taken up the practice, believing it to have sufficient scientific proof. And it is absolutely free! I'd also recommend the documentary called: The Grounded by Steve Kroschel.

On YouTube - *The Grounded* by Steve Krosche
https://youtu.be/cRW0XO2xWn4

Why Go Barefoot
By Stephen T. Sinatra, M.D., F.A.C.C., F.A.C.N., C.N.S., C.B.T.

I go barefoot whenever I can. Why? I love the way it feels, and I know it's better for my body because that's how I was made to walk (not in shoes). But most importantly, because I want my dose of vitamins G and D. When you are outside walking, you can get vitamin D from sunshine. Additionally, you can also get a dose of what I call "vitamin G." G stands for the ground, and vitamin G refers to the natural, gentle electric charge on the Earth's surface.

Find yourself a grassy yard or a grassy park. Better yet, if you are near the beach, stroll along the cool, wet sand as the ocean laps at your feet. If you have any pain or stress when you start out, I guarantee you're going to feel better after a half-hour or hour of walking barefoot. Sitting barefoot, with your feet planted on the ground, is also good (I just prefer walking because of all the health benefits associated with exercise).

"There's something special – almost spiritual, even – about touching the earth. Let's say you've had a challenging day at work. You come home. What's the first thing you do? Take off your shoes, right? When you are barefoot outdoors, something special happens. You feel the ground and suddenly all your anxiety dissipates."

Benefits of Going Barefoot

In today's world, people are largely disconnected from the Earth's energy. Lifestyle changes, including the widespread use of insulating rubber, or plastic-soled shoes, have disconnected us from the energy in the ground, and, of course, we no longer sleep on the ground as in times past. This physical disconnect may actually be an unrecognized cause of inflammation, pain, fatigue, stress, and poor sleep. By reconnecting to the earth, many common symptoms are often relieved and even eliminated: people sleep better, they are more energized, and they feel better.

Transference of the planet's natural, subtle electric energy into your feet and throughout your body is a process known as *Earthing*, or grounding, and is a subject of great interest to me. I co-authored a book titled: *Barefoot Walking* by Michael Sandler and Jessica Lee and have contributed to studies showing that the Earth's energy has a profound nurturing effect on the body.

The potential benefits on the whole body and the aging process are massive. Medically, this is a big deal – a major discovery!

Sandler and Lee mention other, more structure-related benefits of going barefoot in their book. Basically, shoes make our feet conform to their shoe design agendas. Without such agendas, our feet are free to strike the ground as they are designed to do, a biomechanical effect that ultimately means less wear and tear on our bodies. When we rely on shoes to stabilize and support our feet, we don't use our foot muscles. Going barefoot can help us improve our foot strength and stability.

Additionally, walking can result in improved balance due to enhanced signalling from the nerve endings on the bottom of the feet responding more naturally to the ground. Stimulating nerve endings of the feet can also help reduce blood pressure, lower anxiety levels, and boost the immune system.

Do we need any more reason to get outside and go barefoot?

The research on grounding, along with testimonials from all over the world from people who have read the Earthing book, provides intriguing evidence of significant physiological shifts and a healthier functioning body. Anyone can experience such benefits from going barefoot outdoors!

If you live in a colder climate, or just can't spend much time outdoors, you can still tap into the Earth's beneficial energy by using "barefoot substitutes" indoors – special conductive bed sheets, floor mats, and body bands connected by a wire to the ground. You can use these systems while sleeping, working, and relaxing. So, kick off your shoes, walk barefoot, get grounded indoors, and reconnect to Mother Earth!

References & Links:

Grounding-Earthing - from Dr. Stephen Sinatra - *Top Reasons to Go Barefoot this Summer:*
https://heartmdinstitute.com/alternative-medicine-top-reasons-to-go-barefoot-this-summer/
The Expressive Writing Technique - Pennebaker:
https://www.youtube.com/watch?v=XsHIV9PxAV4
Nick & Jessica Ortner EFT: www.thetappingsolution.com
Julie Schiffman EFT: http://eft.mercola.com/
Gene Monterastelli EFT: http://monterastelli.com/
Patricia Carrington Cancer & EFT:
https://patcarrington.com/diagnosis-cancer-how-eft-can-help-arti-cle-2/
Lissa Rankin's Book: Mind Over Medicine:
http://mindovermedicinebook.com/
Meditation Blog-Live and Dare: http://liveanddare.com/benefits-of-meditation/
Time Magazine:
http//heartland.time.com/2010/12/09/mind-over-matter-can-zen-meditation-help-you-forget-about-pain/
NCBI:
http://www.ncbi.nih.gov/pmc/articles/pmc3090218/
David Lynch Foundation:
http://www.davidlynchfoundation.org/university-of-california-at-ir-vine.html
Clint Ober - *Earthing: The Most Important Health Discovery Ever!* (Second Edition) https://amzn.to/33TNd8A

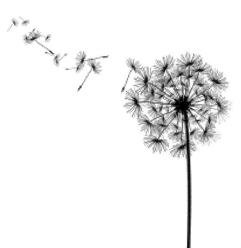

9.   Charles Scopoletti

Heaven Can Wait

Charlie Scopoletti possesses wisdom far beyond his years. His ability to listen, communicate and weave lyrics into the fabric of life are his gifts to the world. Cancer gave him his life's work. Through the music he composes, you come to appreciate his compassionate nature and commitment to living an inspired life. Charlie faced cancer twice; in both instances, music saved him

Please give a warm welcome to Charlie Scopoletti...

Charlie...

My path with cancer is an interesting one because I was diagnosed at two distinct times of my life. Hodgkin's Lymphoma when I was ten. At thirty, I was diagnosed with thyroid cancer; they said it was directly related to cancer treatment as a child.

Cancer as a ten-year-old was an entirely different kind of experience. You're told what to do, where to go and what therapies you'll be undergoing. This was in 1985 and cancer was not at the forefront of the media or fundraising efforts. I was just sick, that's all I knew. I now recognize, because of my experiences as a child with cancer, it helped shape and form the very foundations of my life. These changes came about through the love, kindness, and support of my family, friends, strangers, and the newly formed cancer foundations that were all being relayed to me at an impressionable time in my life. Because of cancer, as a ten your old, I came to appreciate the healing capability of music.

Every Thursday was music day at the hospital. It began with my parents, taking me to the music room in the basement of the hospital hoping to distract me from the nausea of chemo or exhaustion of radiation. In a few weeks, I was the one pleading to be taken there. They were concerned for my wellbeing saying, "No, Charlie, you've just had your treatment, you're not going to feel well." I'd beg, as only a ten-year-old boy can: "I wanna go, I wanna go, I wanna go!"

It was while I was banging on the drums or playing any other instrument, that I'd forget about having cancer. While playing music, I was a healthy normal boy again: no chemo, no radiation, no tumour. The minute the class ended, the side-effects of treatment came rushing back. I'd turn to my mom and say, "I don't feel well."

The music seed was planted as both entertainment and escape, and I would soon discover that the lessons cancer taught me were quietly building the bedrock for my adult life.

For a time, after returning to my then ten-year-old world, I was known as that *kid who had cancer*. Some students were cruel; teasing or bullying me because I'd gained a lot of weight and lost my hair. On the positive side, there were also these amazing kids, some who I never even knew, they would stick up for me. Fortunately, I never felt a personal attachment to cancer, I was heavy into music, acting and I played many sports. Eventually, the positives in my life washed away the cancer label. I was shy talking about cancer, I didn't feel the need to discuss it, I was happy and moving on.

I'm not sure if it was from having cancer or just my personality, but I've always been a positive person. I never liked any sort of confrontation, my sister used to call me Switzerland because I'd always keep the peace in the family or with my friends. In sports I was the captain of the team, always trying to keep everyone's spirits high. I have an encouraging will inside of me; it's grown over time because I've come to understand where it's all coming from and, also the good that comes of it, for the other person and in turn for me.

Music has grown into a career and it's the main driving force in my life. I'm involved in the creative process of performing, composing or writing every day. That shy 10-year-old found an escape in music, all these years later I have the opportunity to help others experience the healing benefits of music. Music has never stopped giving.

Fast forward twenty years. As a direct result of the treatment for Hodgkin's Lymphoma, I developed thyroid cancer at thirty. It was upsetting because, at that point in my life, I was just getting into healthy living. In all those years, no one told me that I might want to watch out for secondary cancer or even that it was a possibility. Had I known the risks I would have added a healthy regime many years earlier.

The discovery of thyroid cancer was all-encompassing. It was at that time my best friend was dying of a brain tumour. She was thirty years old as well. It signified another transition between life, health, and music. When I received the second diagnosis, my response to the doctor was, "Whatever...what do we have to do? Take it out? If that's my option, then that's what I'm going to do, but I'm in control this time." I added, "I'm doing all the things I love, and I don't intend on this stopping me. I'm right in the middle of touring. As a matter of fact, I have a gig next week and I WILL be performing."

I was upset at the recurrence as well as not being told that the treatment for cancer gave me secondary cancer. The doctor said, "You're going to be too tired after surgery." My response, "I'll heal...how soon can I be released and if I go to my gig, will I hurt myself?" He said, "No, you're not going to hurt yourself; you can go, but I'm telling you, you're not going to want to." He added, "All your hormones are gone, you won't have any energy." I didn't care. I was in a fierce mindset. I had friends pick me up and literally carry me to my performance. They sat me on the stool, and I played my concert.

After the second diagnosis of cancer and my best friend passing away, my life became focused. I'm now conscious of the delicacy of life. How precious and how important it is to honour all of life. I wake up each day and commit to:

- ✓ Connecting with my truth
- ✓ Giving to others
- ✓ Offering my message through music

✓ Aligning with my soul's purpose

For me, truth is important. So important in fact that I named my first album *Truth*.

Naturally, people ask me, "What is truth?" My answer is always, "Truth can hold so many meanings. Everyone holds a different universal truth."

For me, truth is *when your dream aligns with your soul's purpose.*

I believe we go after our dreams because that's what we were told to do, or that's what we think we should do. Often when we reach that dream, we realize it's simply not satisfying. Our dream isn't what we expected. The reason for this is because what we're doing with our lives is not in alignment with our purpose. I thought playing music was everything, yet there was a piece missing. I couldn't figure it out. I'd do certain gigs and say, "Wow that was awesome, it felt great, but there has to be more". It wasn't until I started opening up and speaking about my cancer, about my survival and how I've been living straight on, facing things and not letting anything affect me – it was then that I felt a shift inside me.

Opening my heart and myself to other people, being vulnerable – not just through my music but with my words through sharing my story, was the missing piece. It's always been easy for me to write a song and give it out to my audience. But, actually speaking and opening myself up in front of people, saying, "This is me, this is authentically me, this is what my story is."– not until I was wide open, did I feel that alignment with my dream and my purpose. It was then I connected with my truth.

For instance, with the song *Heaven Can Wait*: I wrote it for my parents and my two sisters from the perspective of what I was going through at a critical point in my healing. I knew I was going to be ok no matter what. Whether things got worse or things got better, I'd resolved with myself that I was going to be ok.

I'd lived a good life and I was ready for whatever life had in store for me.

It's difficult to watch your mother, father and sisters be so fearful, to have no control over cancer. Because it was such a difficult thing to witness, I wrote the song *Heaven Can Wait* for them. I needed to tell my family that my love is here to stay, my spirit is always here, so no worries. For me, music has facilitated my healing, first as a ten-year-old in the hospital music room and now, decades later, through my lyrics, my concerts and helping others. Music holds my truth.

These creative forces come out to write these songs. During my concerts, not everyone knows my history, I share a little story on how I wrote the song, but now I'm trying to take it to a deeper level. I inject my experiences behind the songs, really share with my audience what I believe to be true about living life in the moment. By sharing my story of living the best person I can be, really living my truth, it helps me evolve and stay focused too. I believe it's important to not let the days go by wishing to be doing something else with your life. Really hone in on what your truth is, and working on getting there. I'm evolving and growing every day too. If it affects and changes someone in the audience, that's awesome.

At times I need a dose of my own positive medicine. It's been interesting in the last couple of years since they removed my thyroid. I've been on a roller coaster physically; the medicine that

I take doesn't absorb into my body. For the past 8 years, I've been tired all the time. The thyroid gland is commonly referred to as 'your body's gas pedal', and I'm constantly running on fumes. I have to carry on with life regardless of how I'm feeling. When the doctors measure my thyroid levels, they wonder how I function. Everything has an up and a down, low energy has been my biggest challenge.

Once in a while, it's ok to be down. I just accept myself and say, "I'm not going to be the positive one today."

I get into a place where I'm at ease with my bad day. I sit on the couch and watch TV. I accept it, let it work through me and usually, it's gone the next day. I find the more I fight it, complain, worry about not getting things done, the more that low feeling lasts. For the most part, I do what works for me, in order to stay out of it. If I know I'm on the verge of having a bad day, I turn it around by absorbing as much positivity as I can. I watch an inspiring show, read a book, learn something new, or listen to a motivational radio program on Hay House.

I know bad times end, and the upside is definitely my music, my speaking engagements, and my audience. It's a great feeling when I put out a song and a random audience member or someone who recognizes me at an event tells me that my music or lyrics changed their life. That's a powerful motivator to continue. Every live performance I give, I get to see how my music and music in general, has a positive influence on people.

In the last couple of years after I started opening up to people, sharing that side of my life at my concerts or fundraisers, I see firsthand how I can make a difference. Imagine how rewarding it is to receive an email from another ten-year-old, thanking me because my story gave them hope. You just can't beat that. Giving to others restores the energy I lost with my thyroid cancer.

I've been fortunate to have been welcomed into several fantastic cancer organizations with supportive, compassionate individuals. Think about the number of people going through cancer, those who are surviving cancer, as well as the family and friends who know someone who's been touched by cancer.

Being a survivor and an artist I'm in a unique position. I can advocate for, entertain, and inspire people in ways that are both personal and social. The cancer community is such a positive group of people. Everywhere I go, everyone I meet, the events I'm asked to play for or speak at, the people associated with them become an extension of my family.

We've never met, then we talk on the phone or e-mail and instantly I feel like I know them. We have an immediate connection; the power they speak with goes straight to my heart. Eventually, we meet and we're like family. With some, I won't see them until the next big fundraiser and yet I receive emails saying "Hi" or "I'm checking you out on YouTube, see what you're up to. I miss you and I love you."

Cancer has the ability to alter how a person experiences life. I believe for some people who go through it, they resolve themselves to be ok with cancer. Whether they are a survivor, loved one or close friend. And for others, when they lose someone there is so much power, so much love that can come out of it. Because I've experienced all sides of it, they instantly understand I've been where they are. I've felt the loss of someone, and I've lived through the treatment. When we find each other, it's a strong, lovely exchange. If I didn't believe that my voice matters, I wouldn't open up and talk about it, I'd just go on about my life.

For me, cancer doesn't hold any significant weight. Cancer is part of who I am, it doesn't affect me negatively. That's the reason why it's easy for me to speak about and be around cancer patients, or simply to talk straight about cancer. I know in my heart there's hope. I know they can get through it one way or another and if they don't heal physically, I hope they can resolve themselves on how to live their lives in order to be happy until the end.

My best friend who died at 30 was one of those positive people who was happy till the end, teaching people how to be compassionate. She was giving to others, she worried about me and wanted to know if I was ok. She was caring until the end. This is the beautiful side of cancer.

I see cancer as a path. For some, they just don't know how to get to a better place.

All you can do is show them your love and hope they feel it on some level. I'm where I need to be, doing what I'm passionate about.

For now...

Heaven can wait

CHARLIE SCOPOLETTI:
http://www.charliescopoletti.com/music

YOUTUBE - Heaven Can Wait - Charlie Scopoletti:
https://youtube.com/watch?v=plzizyo5ohk

Heaven Can Wait – AppleMusic
https://music.apple.com/us/album/heaven-can-wait/id498071489?i=498071500

Hay Hours Radio
https://hayhouseradio.com/#!/

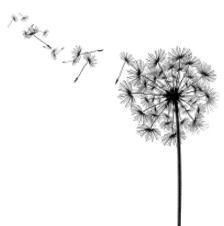

Four Therapeutic Principles for Healing

During chemo and radiation treatment, 10-year-old Charlie Scopoletti experienced the healing outcome that Music Therapy often produces. A sick little boy eagerly banging on drums and strumming a guitar in the basement of the hospital. The therapeutic benefits of music allowed him to access a place of happiness & truth. In music, Charlie found his life's work, his passion, and the curative benefits of giving back. I believe every person has a Happiness Key; Charlie found his through music. It continues to flourish and heal not only in him personally, but the audiences and cancer patients he touches with his unique brand of happiness.

Principle #1 - Music Therapy

The notion that music has the capacity to heal is as ancient as the writings of Aristotle and Plato. The 20th-century profession of Music Therapy formally began after World War I and World War II when community musicians of all types, both amateur and

144

professional, went to veterans' hospitals around the country to play for the thousands of veterans suffering both physical and emotional trauma from the war. The patients' notable physical and emotional responses to music, led the doctors and nurses to request the hiring of musicians by the hospitals. Today there are certified Music Therapy associations in over thirty countries around the globe.

Music has allowed Charlie to stay connected to the range of emotions he identified with as a child and because of those positive experiences, he continues to pay homage to the curative effects through his music. From the joyous, playful ones to the deeply emotional lyrics where his truth resides. He has released two albums titled: TRUTH, and TODAY IS THE DAY.

For Charlie, evidence of Music Therapy's benefits isn't found in a research study – he's living proof of its potential. Through his love of music and the determined man he is, Charlie Scopoletti turned two seemingly negative diagnoses into uplifting lifework. Music paved the way, and he continues to walk this path. Charlie is careful to note that being happy continuously isn't a realistic goal. Honouring the variety and diversity of our personality has health benefits. Without contrast, both creativity life and life overall would be monotone and uneventful. Even continuous elation gets boring after a while. The upswing and downswing in life are similar to the notes of music. You rise and fall, moments of pause and moments of elation. This is one of the reasons our bodies love music, it's diverse and honouring of each inflection. The variations are all vital to the harmony of life and the harmony of a song.

Why people with cancer or chronic illness use imagination and music therapy:
One of the main reasons to use music or imagination therapy

is because it makes you feel better. When you feel better; pain, anxiety, depression, and sickness are lessened.

Music Therapy and using one's imagination can be a safe place for people to explore fear, anxiety, anger, and the range of emotional responses to living with cancer or chronic illness.

Research into music therapy in cancer care:
It's important to note that music therapy cannot cure, treat or prevent any type of disease, including cancer. But some research shows that music therapy can help people with cancer reduce their anxiety. It can also help to improve the quality of life and reduce symptoms and side effects.

We don't yet know about all the ways music can affect the body. But we do know that when music therapy is used in the right way for each person, it can help them to feel better.

Music therapy researchers are increasingly turning their attention to best practices, such as the randomized trial reported from a group at Indiana University. The study tested a specific music therapy intervention, Therapeutic Music Video (TMV), which is designed to improve resilience in adolescent and young adult patients undergoing stem cell transplantation. A total of 113 patients aged 11 to 24 undergoing stem cell transplantation for cancer were randomly assigned to a TMV intervention group or a control group that received audiobooks.

Participants completed six sessions over three weeks. The TMV group demonstrated significantly better measures of courageous coping, social integration, and family environment. Study results support the use of a music-based intervention delivered by a music therapist to help adolescents and young adults positively cope with high-risk, high-intensity cancer treatments.

Investigators in Southern Taiwan studied the effects of music therapy and verbal relaxation on anxiety in outpatients receiving chemotherapy. They randomly assigned 98 patients into three groups: music therapy, verbally guided relaxation, and standard care. Efficacy was measured using the Spielberger State-Trait Anxiety Instrument, Emotional Visual Analog Scale, and three biobehavioral indicators (skin temperature, heart rate, and consciousness level) measured during and after chemotherapy. The researchers found that music therapy had a greater positive effect on post-chemotherapy anxiety than did verbal relaxation or control groups. Patients with high baseline anxiety receiving music therapy had a greater drop in post-chemotherapy anxiety than did those with a predefined "normal" state of anxiety in a subset analysis.

Palliative care teams frequently include music therapists as part of a multidisciplinary approach to the treatment of pain. Researchers at University Hospitals Case Medical Center found that a single music therapy intervention incorporating therapist-guided relaxation and live music effectively lowered pain in palliative care patients. In this study, 200 in-patients were randomly assigned to standard care and with versus without music therapy. The pain was assessed using a numeric rating scale as the primary outcome and the Functional Pain Scale as a secondary outcome. The Face, Legs, Activity, Cry, Consolability (FLACC) scale was also applied as a secondary outcome. Significantly greater decreases in both pain measure scores were seen in the music therapy group; scores did not differ between study groups per the third scale.

Principle #2 - Too Much of a Good Thing

A recent inquiry at UC Berkeley suggests that diversity of emotional experience, described as a rich palette that dynamically spans joy, sadness, love, and anger is more closely linked to happiness and overall health than the common myth that happiness equals a perpetual state of enthusiasm and cheer. Whatever the case, cultivating self-awareness and allowing yourself to express your authentic emotions can be beneficial.

Branch out of your routine and do something new that might make you feel awe or pride; in tough situations, allow yourself to feel shame, or guilt or jealousy rather than what you "should" feel. The idea that wellbeing isn't about being cheerful all the time and avoiding sadness like the plague isn't new to happiness researchers. For example, an October 2012 study found that it might be better for our overall happiness to feel emotions like anger at appropriate times, rather than seeking happiness no matter the situation.

Attempting to hijack emotions into being steady and in control, can backfire on us. Our inner pilot light inherently knows diversity in our feelings gives us perspective. It helps us appreciate when authentic joy is present, allowing one to become accepting and mindful when sadness or fear blankets us. Our emotional body knows when we need to heal, and when we need to slow down and listen.

This is not to imply that you should stay stuck in fear, sadness, or even joy, but rather that authenticity and truth opens you to your natural ease and flow. There will be days when you need to get yourself out of bed, force a smile and keep unsettling feelings to yourself. Making a habit of being too positive or stuck in a pity-party will never serve you or the ultimate goal of healing.

A study by UC Riverside's Sonja Lyubomirsky showed that it might even be possible to gratitude journal too much, losing gratitude's positive effects in the bore of a routine.

Too much of even the good in life is unhealthy and unnatural. The *Key to Happiness*, and a rich, full life is diversity. Not only diversity in your day to day activities, thoughts, and experiences, but through accepting the fullness of your emotions during stressful times in your life.

Cultivating emotional diversity through music, creativity, altruism, compassion, forgiveness, empathy, gratitude, awe, happiness, and social connection, are possible keys to focus on in an attempt to achieve overall wellbeing. As a caveat here, go easy on yourself when you're experiencing a bad day. Be as kind to yourself as you would to a child or friend who's going through similar challenges. One effective practice I've discovered through my research is often referred to as Active Imagination.

Principle #3 – Active Imagination

This practice is used in Jungian Psychology to bridge the gap between the conscious and unconscious mind. As unlikely as this may sound from the perspective of a patient, cancer holds keys to how you can live a life of contentment and authenticity, as was by every person interviewed for this book and countless others whose experiences mirrored those interviewed.

In the stripping away of your health and security, you find yourself steeped in the uncomfortable arms of vulnerability. Behind cancer's unsolicited lessons, you have a unique opportunity to discover your own truth.

To start the practice of *Active Imagination*, dig deep into the recesses of your memories for a time in life when you felt satisfied, unaffected and free of day to day obstacles. Charlie Scopoletti found his buoyant, carefree self through music.

Go back to an event or place in your life when time seemed to evaporate and even if it was physically or emotionally challenging, you felt you were in a state of flow.

Imagine a time when you were a child, teenager, young adult or a more recent time.

If you can't access a happy memory, ask for help from a family member or friend. In times of stress, it can often take the perspective of those closest to us, to trigger carefree memories.

For others, it is possible to have never experienced fulfillment on any significant or memorable level. If this is you, the search needs to focus on moments in life, where you *think* you could have experienced contentment had conditions and circumstances worked in your favour. If you find yourself struggling to locate this happy place, imagine what you think will make you happy, experiment with dreams and ideas, ask those who know you best if they remember a time when you were happy and seemed to have less stress.

I call this your *feel-good-place*, however, feel free to use whatever wording best describes the feeling for you.

Delve into the why and how of these positive moments in your life. Everyone has their own set of criteria for contentment. For you, joy may come through getting still. Others prefer being surrounded by action or activity. It might involve listening to your favourite music or even planning an event or a special vacation.

For those of you who are similar to Charlie Scopoletti, happiness accumulates through giving back to your community by volunteering, motivating or creating joy in the lives of others. There's something to be said for the delight that comes through sharing time with friends, family or colleagues. Active participation in the lives of the people you care about, unconsciously nourishes those relationships, in turn helping your physical, emotional and mental acuity.

Once you've located this *feel-good place*, figure out where in your body you experience it. Pleasant experiences are often deeply rooted in your mind, your body or for some individuals in both regions.

I experience joy in my heart and fear in my solar plexus (belly). Are you able to locate where you feel emotion? If you're having trouble, wait for the next time you experience joy, love or contentment. Where do you feel it?

If you can't find the good, then figure out where you feel fear or even anger. Where in your body does it show up? Sometimes it helps to locate the negative in order to know how an emotion feels in your body. You will have a similar, yet, positive reaction to pleasant emotions. We're doing this in order to embody the emotions of happiness. It's always easier to get in touch with how our bodies respond to emotions when we know where they typically show up.

Once we know this, we can give ourselves physical cues, such as touching or patting those parts of our bodies that are the source of positive emotion. It's a quick way to accelerate or calm our physical reactions. For this process, we are trying to ignite the *feel-good-place* and remember, in turn triggering joy, happiness, bliss.

Take some time to write these memories down in as much detail as possible. If writing isn't convenient, simply imagine yourself in that happy place. Again, go into as much detail as you can. Play it out in your imagination as if you were directing a movie. Where were you, who was with you, what time of year, what you were wearing, recall any scents, what were you eating, were you standing, driving, on vacation, alone, at a party? Details are the keys to success when attempting to recreate positive memories.

Through examining what attracts you to these moments of bliss, you are forming the vital first step of peeling back the layers that cultivate joy and happiness. It's in the stripping away of these emotional layers that your contented self comes into view, then the real work begins.

As Charlie Scopoletti explained in Chapter 7, *Heaven Can Wait*, once you discover what works for you and brings contentment to your life, you are given clues as to what elements are required for you to easily access those happy emotions. As you work this mental muscle, then you can quickly return to this *feel-good-place* in your body and spark the imagination. With practice, you'll have easier access when the challenges of illness and treatment leave you feeling vulnerable and alone.

The power of imagination can transport you to this *feel-good-place*. With consistent training of your optimistic imagination, your mind, causes your body to react comparably to the moment that pleasing event initially took place. It's a memory hack that your mind, body, and cells, are unable to interpret the difference between actually experiencing it or remembering it.

Active Imagining is a process of closing the gap between past positive experiences. Keep in mind, the same experience takes place with a fearful or adverse event in your life. Negativity is a powerful emotion and when we replay it in our imagination, it then becomes a downhill spiral of feelings emotions and physical symptoms.

When you attach emotions to this practice, it has the potential to change lives and influence your overall wellbeing. When you're happy and contented, your body has the opportunity to heal physically, emotionally and spiritually. It naturally lowers the experience of being smothered by fear, anger, sadness or any one of the many damaging emotions residing in our overactive sometimes theatrical minds.

In those moments when you come face to face with a crisis, the critical pieces of the wellbeing puzzle are often lost in the dark folds of fear. Finding those missing pieces has the potential to point you in the direction of your truth. Once unearthed, the real work begins – as Charlie Scopoletti mentioned, even though he was living his dream of being a musician, after each performance, he felt a key piece was missing in his concerts and his life. Through sharing his cancer story, writing and speaking openly about the struggles in his life, the missing pieces that made up his joy and happiness puzzle were realized. Charlie discovered he has three needs: Composing, Performing and Communicating.

Your needs will be unique to you. Once you discover them, you'll be in a position to weave them into the fabric of your life. From this work, you'll open opportunities for expanded joy, happiness and contentment. Under the umbrella of these constructive emotions, healing has a chance to flourish.

Looking at cancer as an *opportunity* to examine where you find joy is an essential component of overall health. Your emotional healing is as urgent as is your physical healing. When you encourage and exercise your mind and body simultaneously, they literally join forces to assist in your recovery. Remember, the mind is in every cell throughout your body. We are made up of over 50 trillion cells. It's a community living inside us, and you're the governing body of those cells. Like all governments, they work best with your full support, attitude, and belief. Similar to your cells on medicine, your physiology and biology are aided by your belief in its effectiveness and the power to heal.

Active Imagination fuels belief. Belief, in turn, allows healing to flow to and through you. Unlocking the path to your happiness and truth begins with a single step.

I guarantee you won't unlock the path on the other side by having more money, the perfect partner, a new baby, ideal home, shiny car, or the ultimate vacation. Happiness and truth are created in the inner workings of how you:

✓ Give Back
✓ Show Up in Your Life
✓ Forgive Mistakes You've Made
✓ Forgive Mistakes of Others
✓ Embrace and Share the Gifts You've Been Given.

Every day, there's a morsel of good hiding in the simple things, even if you can't see it immediately. You may be looking in the wrong direction or noticing all the negatives or giving in to fear as it encompasses you.

Finding a single positive thing about your illness moves you in the direction of improved health and wellness. The truth is, your cancer has something to teach you, it will improve your life and the lives of those around you if you stop resisting, drop the anger and allow cancer to reveal to you what it's here to teach you. I'm not suggesting that this is a time for celebration, giving up on healing, or finding the reasons and action steps toward overcoming it. Looking for positivity in adversity goes deeper than cells and chemo. Think of it as DNA Transformation for the soul, healing you from the inside out.

When Charlie Scopoletti decided to perform in front of an audience a few days after his thyroid surgery, he used willpower and *Active Imagination* to propel himself onto the stage. It was his absolute goal and belief in the strength of music to heal him and others. Nothing stopped him. Not his well-meaning surgeon, the medical facts of thyroid cancer, or his splintered physical body. Music Therapy had taught him that when he played music, the pain diminished, and anything was possible. When Charlie turned to music, his happiness and truth bubbled to the surface. It didn't change the pain, it changed his experience of pain. Try *Active Imagination* for yourself and experience the power of your own mind.

Principle #4 - Mental Training Exercise
In the book *Psycho-Cybernetics*, author Dr. Maxwell Maltz (1960) gives examples of the limitations of those who've influenced us from childhood: schools, families, cultures, and workplace environments into believing non-truths about society,

our potential, and ourselves. Dr. Maltz gives us a mental training exercise to overcome these limitations.

Truth Determines Action and Behaviour- by Dr. Mathew Maltz (1960)

The human brain and nervous system are engineered to react automatically and appropriately to the problems and challenges in the environment. For example, a man does not need to stop and think that that self-survival requires that he run if he meets a grizzly bear on a trail. He does not need to decide to become afraid.

The fear response is both automatic and appropriate. First, it makes him want to flee. The fear then triggers bodily mechanisms that "soup up" his muscles so that he can run faster than he has ever run before. His heartbeat is quickened. Adrenaline, a powerful muscle stimulant, is poured into the bloodstream. All bodily functions not necessary to running are shut down. The stomach stops working, and all available blood is sent to the muscles. Breathing is much faster and the oxygen supply to the muscles is increased manifold.

All this, of course, is nothing new. Most of us learned it in high school. What we have not been so quick to realize, however, is that the brain and nervous system that reacts automatically to the environment is the same brain and nervous system that tells us what the environment is. The reactions of the man meeting the bear are commonly thought of as due to "emotion" rather than to ideas. Yet it was an idea – information received from the outside world and evaluated by the mind that sparked the so-called "emotional reactions."

Thus, it was basically an idea or belief that was the true causative agent, rather than emotion, which came as a result. In short, the man on the trail reacted to what he thought, believed, or imagined the environment to be. The messages brought to us from the environment consist of nerve impulses from the various sense organs. These nerve impulses are decoded, interpreted and evaluated in the brain, and made known to us in the form of ideas or mental images. In the final analysis, it is these mental images that we react to.

Note that I've used the terms thought, believed, and imagined as synonymous. In affecting your entire system, they are the same. You act and feel according to what things are really like, but according to the image your mind holds of what they are like. You have certain mental images of yourself, your world, and the people around you, and you behave as though these images were the truth, the reality, rather than the things they represent.

Suppose, for example, that the man on the trail had not met a real bear, but a movie actor dressed in a bear costume. If he thought and imagined the actor to be a bear, his emotional and nervous reactions would have been exactly the same. Or suppose he met a large shaggy dog, which his fear-ridden imagination mistook for a bear. Again, he would react automatically to what he believed to be true concerning himself and his environment.

It follows that if our ideas and mental images concerning ourselves are distorted or unrealistic, then our reaction to our environment will likewise be inappropriate.

Can these causative factors change?

Certainly: Consider the child raised in a poor family, made up of people who profoundly believe that their unhappy circumstances are the fault of evil rich people and a corrupt government, who constantly program the child with class warfare ideas, and who insist that they just cannot get ahead no matter what they do. This truth may very well *block that person's academic achievement, direct him away from college, have him blindly follow his father to work in the factory or the coal mine. (Well, I show my age with the "coal mine," I suppose.) Yet, even today, the basic path of accepting poverty as a "fact" is prevalent in many, many people. But how does one person rise out of a background to become a highly successful entrepreneur, for example?*

Through books he's exposed to, people he sees on television, the influence of a mentor, life experiences — one way or another challenging what he believed to be true, discovering it is based on illusion, and replacing that truth with another truth.

You can change from anything to anything by changing your Happiness & Truth (self-image) *by providing it with a new truth.*

Why Not Imagine Yourself Successful?

Realizing that our own actions, feeling, and behaviour are the result of our own images and beliefs gives us the lever that psychology has always needed for changing personality.

It opens a powerful psychological door to gaining skills, success, and happiness.

Mental pictures offer us an opportunity to practice new traits and attitudes which otherwise we could not do. This is possible because again, your nervous system cannot tell the difference between an actual experience and one that is vividly imagined.

If we picture ourselves performing in a certain manner, it is nearly the same as the actual performance. Mental practice is as powerful as actual practice.

Below, I've listed a visualization exercise by Dr. Maxwell Maltz, author of *Psycho-Cybernetics*. Filtering through entire sections of bookstores and libraries which are devoted to helping you find joy, happiness, and contentment can be overwhelming.

Use caution and your intuition to guide you into awareness of what feels right to you. It is quite possible you will receive advice and literature from well-meaning friends and family. Take time to decide what resonates with you. It's not necessary to read every book, blog, or research study that's sent to you. Be discriminating: the amount of information is overwhelming.

To assist you in acquiring a mental picture of when and where you were in a state of pure joy, try this self-image exercise from the book *Psycho-Cybernetics* by Dr. Maxwell Maltz. It was written in 1960 for business success, however, it's still used and quoted today to help reshape negative patterns that no longer serve us. For the purpose of this chapter, I've added the words "happiness" and "contentment" to the original text of self-image. I'd encourage you to read his expanded explanation and method in his book. You'll find this particular exercise at the end of chapter 3.

MENTAL TRAINING EXERCISE

Your present image of happiness & truth (self-image) was built from your own imagination: pictures of yourself in the past, which grew out of interpretations and evaluations you learned through experience. "Whether we realize it or not, each of us carries with us a mental blueprint or picture of ourselves...it has been built up from our own beliefs about ourselves. But most of these beliefs about ourselves have unconsciously been formed from our past experiences, our successes and failures, our humiliations, our triumphs, and the way other people have reacted to us, especially in early childhood."

Keep in mind, you are to use the same method to build an adequate self-image of happiness and contentment that you previously used to build an inadequate one. Set aside a period of 30 minutes each day where you can be alone and undisturbed. Relax and make yourself as comfortable as possible. Now close your eyes and exercise your imagination.

Many people find they get better results if they imagine themselves sitting before a large motion-picture screen and imagine that they are seeing a motion picture of themselves. The important thing is to make these pictures as vivid and as detailed as possible. You want your mental pictures to approximate actual experience as much as possible. The way to do this is to pay attention to small details: sights, sounds, and objects in your imagined environment. Details of the imagined environment are all important in this exercise because, for all practical purposes, you are creating a practice experience. And if the imagination is vivid enough and detailed enough, your imagination practice is equivalent to an actual experience, insofar as your nervous system is concerned.

The next important thing to remember is that during these 30 minutes you see yourself acting and reacting appropriately, success-fully, ideally. It doesn't matter how you acted yesterday. You do not need to try to have faith you will act in an ideal way tomorrow. Your nervous system will take care of that in time if you continue to practice. See yourself acting, feeling, being as you want to be. Do not say to yourself, "I am going to act this way tomorrow." Just say to yourself, "I am going to imagine myself acting this way now, for 30 minutes today." Imagine how you would feel if you were already the sort of personality you want to be.

As a patient, if you have been shy and timid, unable to advocate for your own health needs, see yourself speaking with your doctors and nurses, asking relevant questions and concerns with ease and poise, and feeling strong because of it. If you have been fearful and anxious in medical situations, see yourself acting calmly and deliberately, acting with courage and feeling expansive and confident because you are able to express yourself with respect and knowledge. If you are unable to find a time in your life where you were happy, healthy, and confidant, build an image of a time where you were. A time when you said and did all the right things and the day belonged to you.

This exercise builds new "memories" or stored data into your mid-brain and central nervous system. It builds a new image of self. After practicing it for a time, you will be surprised to find yourself "acting differently," more or less automatically and spontaneously, without trying. This is as it should be. You do not need to take thought, or try, or make an effort now in order to feel ineffective and act inadequately. Your present inadequate feeling and doing are automatic and spontaneous, because of the memories, real and imagined you have built into your automatic mechanism. You will find it will work just as automatically upon positive thoughts and experiences as upon negative ones.

Step One: Take a pad and pen and write out a brief outline or description of the mental movie you intend to construct, experiment with, develop, and view in the theatre in the mind.

Step Two: Set aside 30 minutes a day, preferably at the same time each day, to find a quiet, private place. Relax, close your eyes, enter your theatre, and begin playing, editing, and replaying your movie.

Step Three: Gradually "massage" your movie so that its "star" (you) performs exactly as you desire and achieves the experience and results you desire. Strive to arrive at this point within the first 10 days.

Step Four: *The remaining 11 days, play and enjoy that movie repeatedly, without change.*

Quotes by Maxwell Maltz:

> "*Human beings always act, feel and perform in accordance with what they imagine to be true about themselves and their environment.*"
>
> "*I have found that one of the most common causes of unhappiness among my patients is that they are attempting to live their lives on the deferred payment plan. They do not live, nor do they enjoy life now, but wait for some future event or occurrence. They will be happy when (they are healthy), when they get married, when they get a better job, when they get the house paid for, when they get the children through college, when they have completed some task or won some victory. Invariably, they are disappointed.*
>
> *Happiness is a mental habit, a mental attitude, and if it is not learned and practiced in the present it is never experienced. It cannot be made contingent on solving some external problem. When one problem is solved, another appears to take its place. Life is a series of problems. If you are to be happy at all, you must BE HAPPY - period! Not happy because of.*"

Sources

Journal of Music Therapy and Music Perspectives:
http://mtp.oxfordjournals.com

Too Much of a Good Thing:
https://greatergood.berkeley.edu/article/item/variety_is_the_spice_of_emotional_life

The New Psycho-Cybernetics:
https://www.amazon.com/New-Psycho-Cybernetics-Maxwell-Maltz/dp/0735202850

Cancer Research UK:
http://www.cancerresearchuk.org/about-cancer/cancer-in-general/treatment/complementary-alternative-therapies/individual-therapies/music

Karen Popkin, LCAT, MT-BC, HPMT:
http://www.ascopost.com/issues/september-15-2014/the-role-of-music-therapy-in-cancer-care

PubMed=Chemo & Music Therapy:
Lin MF, Hsieh YJ, Hsu YY, et al: A randomized controlled trial of the effect of music therapy and verbal relaxation on chemotherapy-induced anxiety. J Clin Nursing 20:988-999, 2011.

Music Therapy for Pain Management:
Gutgsell KJ, Schluchter M, Margevicius S, et al:
Music therapy reduces pain in palliative care patients: A randomized controlled trial. J Pain Symptom Manage 45:822-831, 2013.

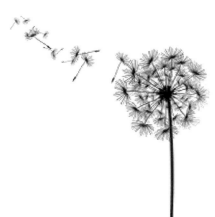

11. Barbara Marx Hubbard

Cancer is the body's panicked effort to grow without a plan

To the world, Barbara Marx Hubbard is known as "The Mother of Conscious Evolution." At 89 she possesses a youthful beauty, infectious laugh, and innate wisdom. Barbara is a compelling passionate leader in the field of consciousness. After a diagnosis of Chronic Lymphocytic Leukaemia at the age of 74, the woman and conscious leader stepped into the predominantly allopathic world of cancer. Considering her history in teaching and living consciousness, it's not surprising Barbara chose integrative and non-traditional cancer treatments. Out of this experience a new and exciting field of growth for us all.

Barbara's transformational journey with cancer began 24 years earlier when she had an experience to which she was summoned to: Step into her life's purpose or die!

Barbara...

I was cleaning out my basement, which is a perfect little metaphor for what was about to be revealed. In my head, I heard the words, "Would you like to die?"

I was shocked as I had no suicidal thoughts, my response was a definitive, "NO." The inner voice inquired, 'Would you like to get cancer, or would you like to rejuvenate?' I responded, "I didn't know I had a choice, obviously I would like to rejuvenate."

What I heard next would alter the course of my life:

"Cancer is the body's panicked effort to grow without a plan; rejuvenation occurs when you say yes to the deeper plan of your being, life purpose or vocation."

I want to make it clear that this *Does Not* mean everyone without a plan, purpose or vocation, will get cancer. The voice was directed to me personally.

In that moment, at the age of 50, standing in my basement, I made a strong and specific declaration:

"I want to rejuvenate and not get cancer. Therefore, I am dedicated to a deeper understanding of the plan of my being."

I went full out for the next 14 years, I focused on evolving and sharing my knowledge. As the mother of five children, I was going through many shifts. It became clear to me, menopause itself was a time for deeper discovery of the planetary being. I followed this conviction without reservation and continued moving in the direction of my life's purpose. For me, it included running for vice president, writing books, teaching classes, even attempting to rent a space rocket. I was fully living my purpose.

As so often happens in life, I lost impulse and my life direction. I was facing a temporary decline in commitment to my purpose. I felt I was heading in the right direction however, I wasn't doing it fully. What showed up in early 2003, was a series of sudden illnesses: bronchitis, pneumonia, and appendicitis. I was using meditation and a healthy lifestyle as a way of healing the ailments. Without warning, my appendix ruptured, and I found myself in hospital in a serious health crisis requiring an emergency appendectomy.

When the doctor examined me after surgery, he informed me my blood work showed I had abnormal white blood cells, indicating I had Chronic Lymphocytic Leukaemia. My response was definitive: *"No, I don't...I couldn't possibly have anything like that, that's not true."*

Despite my objections, the fact was, I had cancer. There were decisions to be made about my health and my life's purpose. I discovered that Chronic Lymphocytic Leukaemia is an over-proliferation of abnormal white blood cells. The function of the white blood cell is to protect you. In my case, there were too many inside my body. My white blood cells had an "over-active" sense of urgency of their purpose. I saw this as another perfect metaphor reminding me: *"Cancer is the body's panicked effort to grow without a plan; regeneration occurs when you say yes to the deeper plan of your being."* I was convinced this health crisis was related to the loss of life's purpose.

The doctors told me that as long as the cancer doesn't spike, that is to say, rapidly rise, I'd be OK. They call it a smoking gun. Now we are all living to some degree with a smoking gun. However, mine had a name. Fortunately, it could be measured and monitored. Through additional blood tests, it showed the counts were gradually rising. It was like a slow-motion experience of cancer. I did a lot of things at that time, I had infusions, I had deep cell microscopy – looking under a microscope I was able to witness the white blood cells acting like nasty little varmints, attacking the beautiful red blood cells. I found it fascinating to see the degree of warfare of abnormal white cells *acting with a purpose*, they were urgently attacking the vulnerable red blood cells. It became a metaphor for my own life. Without a focus, our physical, emotional and spiritual systems become prey to that which has an urgency of purpose.

On the level of my work and life's purpose, it took an extreme amount of energy. I felt a little lost and began to move further into the life of being simply a narrator of what I know. I was teaching classes on the internet and having more of a chance to reach out to spread that knowledge. I wasn't living it the way my soul wanted me to though. Simply participating in my life's work wasn't enough, I needed to embody it. Perhaps this lack of commitment was the reason for the illness in the first place. Because of cancer in my life, it continues to teach me and keeps me focused on my higher life purpose.

I'm committed to the message I received: *"Cancer is the body's panicked effort to grow without a plan; regeneration occurs when you say yes to the deeper plan of your being."*

A daunting thought, and please understand I'm not generalizing, I don't believe everyone who gets cancer is without a purpose. In my case it was absolutely true, I did not have a clear life pattern for my bigger life's purpose, I was feeling stuck and urgent. The cancer cells were mirroring how I felt, they were urgent in their work and yet not going the whole way to kill me. They seemed to be stuck too.

Regeneration happens when you have discovered the deeper plan of your being, life's purpose or vocation. Particularly when you are a woman over 50 if you are no longer producing eggs, you are not going to reproduce the species. Either you're going to evolve by giving birth to some greater potential of your inner plan of action, or, as in my case, grow a cancer, in order to get my attention. This understanding was directed to me personally, again I want to emphasize, it does not mean without an inner plan of action, you will get or have cancer.

I made a decision to focus on the deepest work I could, in order to discover my life purpose. I had been on this path, but I felt I didn't know exactly what to do next. Like me, my white blood cells were doing their job attacking the red blood cells, but not completely. It was as if they didn't have a clear understanding of their purpose. I decided to try something out. I would attempt to communicate with my cancer cells through visualization, and informing them:

"Dear white blood cells, I realize you have a lot of growth potential and seeing how you are using your potential without an organized plan, I will do my best to give you a better plan."

The strategy was to rejuvenate me however, these semi-productive cancer cells wouldn't be receptive to my plan for them unless I found the bigger plan of my own life.

My work is a *vocation of destiny*. It's different than a good job, a *vocation of destiny* is something you feel born to do. I feel born to the particular calling of teaching evolving consciousness. With the cancer diagnosis, I now had the impetus to focus all my resources in the direction of my work. To believe in it fully and strive to be in charge of my destiny and in turn the fate of my cancer. It was as if I had to prove to cancer my commitment to myself and my work through believing in and teaching my vocation of destiny. With a total belief in my purpose, I would give cancer a better plan.

In recognition of this need for a higher plan, I knew the planet was in a crisis, I realized that we didn't have a lot of time to change. I identified myself as a cell in the planetary body. I've always felt myself as a member of the planet. I believe I'm on planetary time, not personal time. If the planet was going through a crisis of running out of energy and possible destruction of its environment, I had a role to fulfill as a member of the planet. Not only did I feel it, but I felt its urgency. I believed somehow, I had to do something about our planet. A lot of people feel that way, but in my case, I felt it acutely because of cancer.

Now, this is an important point: the discovery of a plan of your being is discovering your individual plan, not somebody else's. It isn't, "oh well it would be nice to do something, so I'll just figure it out, I'll join this club, or I'll do that." No, you have to find your unique genius code, the one that holds the frequency and energy of your cells. Taking care of your family, working at a job you love, inspiring others, speaking your truth. Whatever it is that gets you excited and open to opportunity for growth.

For me, growth was imperative both for my health and for my cancer. You see, if my cancer was to win, to achieve its higher purpose by killing me, it would have to die along with my body.

A higher plan to grow in the direction of regeneration was the logic I used. I theorized if we all worked together, it was possible to coexist. I didn't go about wishing to destroy the cells, but to give them a lesson in conscious evolution. We have learned from Bruce Lipton's book – *The Biology of Belief,* that our DNA is affected by the consciousness around it and by the membrane that covers each cell. Through his work, I realize I have some effect on my own DNA script. I decided to take it as a real signal to tune into the better part of my plan in order to:

- ✓ See if I could stay alive.
- ✓ Fulfill my life purpose – *this was actually more important to me.*
- ✓ Discover if fulfilling this higher plan had any effect on my regeneration.

That was well over ten years ago, I'm going on 88 and experiencing ever more energy. I have also coined a funny phrase:

"Some people swallow an evolve pill in their mother's milk, they have a tendency to want to evolve."

Others really don't have that tendency, they're not turned on by a deeper life purpose, so when they get to be a certain age they degenerate. When I think about retiring at 65 it's actually ridiculous, given the energy that is in all of us. Then when you consider your life's purpose that energy is even greater.

I wrote a book called *52 Codes for Conscious Evolution* - these 52 codes are guidelines for the universal self.

In addition, I'm working with a small team of people we've named *The Universal Human Pod.* It's fascinating from the point of view of cancer. How it works is: we meet over the phone, once or twice a week. We connect with the Local Self, the Essential Self, the Universal Self, and then the God Self. Which is to say the supreme divine substance of reality. Within this alliance of energies, we are *symbolically* placing our bodies together and we've created a cocoon of light. The *Cocoon of Light* has a membrane using Bruce Lipton's idea. Adopting Dr. Lipton's theory, we are a membrane of a multicellular organism.

We go from the ME to WE to ONE - A multi-human cell. What happens within this cocoon of light when you start accessing all the frequencies of your being and bringing your own body in there, all 50 trillion of your cells are activated and each and every one of those cells is a unique being.

On these *Universal Human Pod* phone conversations, I bring my 50 trillion cells, which still have the degenerative white blood cells moving around, the others in the group have their own health challenges and in the time we've been meeting, we've noticed an acceleration of regeneration.

There is a feeling of oneness, a better description would be the wholeness of another world. The reason being, we are a new *whole system* – by taking all levels of our being, accessing them and then connecting them. In other words, I have my soul's code in my essential self in this pod, everybody else is identifying their *soul's code* in their pod in their life, and our individual *soul codes* are connecting. Through this work, I'm very close to being able to hold that cocoon of light within myself, all the time. It doesn't depend on being on the phone with the others. But it is necessary to repeat it over, and over again.

I call it an Evolutionary Eucharist.

The Catholics have practiced the ritual of the Eucharist for thousands of years, eating the body and blood of Christ. The whole Christian Religion is about symbolically eating the body and blood of Christ. Basically, that is what we are doing in our *Universal*

Human Pod, we are moving it up to the risen body through three channels;

- ✓ The *universal self-bodies* of ourselves
- ✓ The *essential-selves* of ourselves
- ✓ The 50 trillion cells of *ourselves*

We are taking our *whole-selves* into that higher vibration.

All cultures, all traditions, all religions have had versions of the Light Body and considering every religion has had one version or another of their masters being Light Bodies, I began to take it as literally true that everybody who is evolving has access to their own Light Body. All of this is just frequency anyway, that is all we are. When you tap into the higher frequency of your own being, which you could call *Universal Self*.

Universal Self is a little less intimidating than using the term *Light Body*, but it does have the quality of light to it. To give you an example of what I've been doing: I can, at this moment, communicate directly with my cells by saying: *"dearly beloved white cells, this is the larger plan now".*

Medically, I have an oncologist and I take bio-identical hormones. I have blood tests regularly. What has happened is the white blood cells have stabilized or are in remission. I'm not completely cancer-free, I still have more white blood cells and the diagnosis of Chronic Lymphocytic Leukaemia stands, the cancer hasn't gone away, it's just in a holding pattern. I feel that I'm actually regenerating through the act and my belief that I am regenerating. My absolute belief in my own belief is causing this remission of sorts.

In part, I think this remission is due to discovering I have more of a life purpose.

It's not even just communicating with my cells, it's more and more about conscious evolution. It is being the evolving human MYself, with everybody else *being* the evolving human THEM-selves, on our planet earth. Without evolving, we humans will die, or at the very least, the species as we know it will be destroyed. The timing on the planet is much more conducive to me giving my gift of understanding conscious evolution, and for it to be received by a larger audience of readers and enlightened beings. Interestingly I've re-released a book I wrote in 1998 entitled *Conscious Evolution*, and it's actually as relevant today, if not more so, because our planet is more aware than we've ever been.

Not unlike my cancer, my awareness of it has given me greater authority over cancer. I'm taking action steps toward giving my white blood cells a new purpose instead of the other way around.

Evolving humans are in the midst of the planetary shift as Dr. Ervin Laszlo has done in his work on the Akashic Field of science. I believe we are tapping into the Akashic Field and I believe this is a new norm. As Dr. Laszlo explains you have two choices: *"extinction or evolution"*. In other words, cancer is extinction or evolution. I'm in a deep experiment of taking consciously the whole-body into a cocoon of light, which I spoke of earlier, with all the levels of frequency, all the way up to the God-Head, all the way down to the smallest cell in my body.

During this experiment in communication with my cancer cells, I communicate directly with them through dialogue such as; *"White cells: this is your opportunity now, to truly understand the new plan of the evolving human. White cells, wouldn't it be wonderful for you to see that your efforts of over urgency that lead to destruction, could become your own salvation, your own motivation evolved. Dearly beloved white blood cells. It's a simple fact, if you achieve your objective of destroying my healthy cells, you lose your existence, along with me."*

On these *Universal Human Pod* phone conversations, our cocoon of light, with the membrane around us, we raise our-selves up to the highest frequency of our being, for the purpose of embodiment. Not for the purpose of transcendence, for:

- ✓ trans-FORMATION
- ✓ trans-FIGURATION
- ✓ em-BODIMENT
- ✓ in-CARNATION

I say to my white cells: *"dear white cells, look at your opportunity here, wouldn't it be wonderful if you actually were able to fulfill your greater destiny, which would be to evolve into elements of regeneration?"*

For me, it's my white blood cells, for others, some other form of conversation with their DNA script. Educating their cells toward regeneration, longevity, rejuvenation. It's essential for human evolution when each person has access to the plan of their being. So, it's really necessary for the white blood cells to understand rejuvenation here. I find it interesting that statistically, medicine has done a lot of progress with every disease except cancer. Even though there's been a small degree of improvement, it's much less than other diseases.

My insight into this through my research is that it's because cancer is so fundamental to the way the organism exists and evolves. In other words, it is intrinsic to the cell because the cells always replicate and replicate up to a point. If they live a certain length of time, they get errors in their duplication, and cancer becomes almost a way of killing us because we have to die, you were supposed to die. That's the way the plan is so far.

What if the plan itself is changing not only the personal plan of individuals but the plan of the larger population being called to greater wisdom, greater creativity, greater participation in the conscious evolution of humanity? What I'm really saying here is: the evolution of the cancer cell, at the time when random growth and overgrowth is killing the species and people are living longer and longer lives is potentially a call to cancer cells requiring the cells to regenerate and that regeneration may happen by giving us more vitality. That is – if we have more of a sense of pattern and plan, rather than if we don't and in which case you don't continue living.

What if one of the greatest factors is whether or not one has a plan of action internalized to live our purpose or soul's code. Or to know why you're here on this earth, and you know you're not here to just reproduce and die as we were taught so long ago when people didn't live much longer than 55 or 60. Consider how most postmenopausal women in this century are regenerating, rejuvenating.

I have a new word for it, *Regenopause*, it means you are regenerating during the pause, that is IF you have discovered a life purpose or have a vocation of destiny. When you *Regenopause*, as I'm doing, something else starts to happen which is what I call *Supra-Sexual Co-Creation*. Sexuality is joining genes to reproduce, *Supra-Sexuality* is joining genus to evolve oneself, one's work and the world. Nature put joy into sexuality for us to reproduce up to maximum, which it has done and now nature is putting joy into co-creativity, in order to get us to join in order to create. When we join to create, like my friends and I are doing on our *Universal Human Pod* phone conversations, when you place yourself in the cocoon of light, you begin to regenerate, you must because you have more to do.

Nature is very pragmatic, it's not all about beauty and it's certainly not about having wrinkles or not. Nature IS about life pulse, it is life passion. To be, to express, and to create the essence of the divine aspect of God, or your own definition of Higher being. Whatever the word you use for it, it is the evolving God-Head, incarnate.

Cancer really is a call to everyone to evolve, it is a guideline that I use to evolve that is, to be open to everybody. I believe cancer is a signal and evolving is such a positive response to that signal, no matter what happens, for however long anyone has to live. If we didn't have the disease, we wouldn't have the stress required for evolution, because problems are evolutionary drivers, you either go extinct or you evolve.

That's the 13.8-billion-year trend. Through evolution, species go extinct all the time. The only difference is we are conscious of it, that's what conscious evolution is and why it has become conscious in humans. This realization is a huge step forward not only for those of us with cancer – for the evolution of the world, and all of us in it.

Through this evolution, I'm discovering levels of motherhood:

The first level of motherhood was having five children. It could be a career or a marriage, a birthing or creation of some kind.

The second level of motherhood was giving birth to my own unique potential self, a vocation, a life purpose.

The third level of motherhood, I'm coming into right now and it seems to be multidimensional – it's mothering as a whole.

I feel like it's planetary motherhood. I seem to be mothering myself forward toward becoming a universal human. I've always believed we are emerging as a new species and the big shock to find is that we are ALL one of them. Then you begin to do a double take on yourself, and you say: "Is it true, is it really so, am I emerging as this new species?" I'm asking others the same question. I think one of my great pleasures is going to be the question I would like to ask other women especially, "how are you feeling as a whole, where are you on your own personal evolutionary scale?" I want to serve others in my next iteration here, as one going through this change, and going through this is a new norm with humility, with a sense of discovery, rather than someone who knows it all.

What I received in my guidance is that you can't just have one universal pod, you need many, and within that, we have many people joining together. I would like to be a voice for many universal humans to form pods. I would like to be one that helps nurture those pods into the fulfillment of their members and the planet itself. How would the planet evolve except by us evolving, who else is going to do it?

Our culture is afraid of aging, it's been my experience my age helps with this type of evolution. I've realized that though aging you gain authority. This is another big question, "Where on this earth do you find authority?" It's not in any of the places we are used to looking: Politics, Religion, Global Corporations. Where do we find authority?

I'm teaching my cells authority internally and, also where I need to move my own life in the world, and, also to be an authority for anyone who can use me. That is what authorities are for, we are here to give other people authority. My hope is that more and more people feel the authority within themselves. I want others to ask two questions of themselves:

1. Do I feel I have fully accessed my deeper life's purpose?
2. What steps am I willing to take in order to work on achieving that?

Don't do it alone, find one other person with whom to work on finding your deeper life purpose, go into a resonant field, resounding one's love and *higher self, higher mind*. I would like to give that to everybody, then if you feel so called, reach out to others to form communities of people practicing self-evolution through joining as one, as a whole: in these communities there is a new culture.

The call is to help build a new culture, through yourselves and through this dis-ease called cancer.

For additional information visit:
www.BarbaraMarxHubbard.com

At the time this book was being edited Barbara Marx Hubbard passed away April 10, 2019.

The letter below was posted on her website and Facebook page by her friend and business partner Marc Gafni.

Let's Talk About The C Word

Dearest Beloved Friends,

It is with great personal sadness that I share with you that our beloved Barbara has passed into the next world just a few hours ago.

Barbara, you were a blazing light in this world.

The Wild Stallions that moved you were yoked to the evolutionary impulse itself. Evolution was awake as you in Person. Reality delighted in having a Barbara experience.

You felt the ecstatic urgency of the evolutionary impulse moving through you all the time.

You took the pain of depression and turned it into the joy of evolutionary activism.

You took fate and turned it into destiny time and again. You were the greatest Evolutionary Storyteller of our time.

You dreamed of social synergy, of the Peace Room, the Office for the Future, you incarnated a vice-presidential bid, a historic speech at the democratic national convention, the great Foundation for Conscious Evolution, all of these were the vehicles you audaciously manifested for the impulse.

Abraham Maslow, Bucky Fuller, Jonas Salk, and so many more, including this writer, – you charmed us all, you recognized us all, you inspired us, you called us forth with you.

Friends allow me for a moment to be intensely personal. I spoke to Barbara last Friday evening. She was filled with life. We were going over the evolutionary code I had written for evolutionary church the next morning.

Barbara, I called you the next morning. The nurse said you were not well. She held the phone to your ear; you said filled with life, "Marc" ...and that was the last word you spoke. I flew to the hospital to see you right after church – on the next flight – expecting to meet you after the surgery – awake and fully alive. You did not wake up.

It is trite to say but it all happened so fast. I thought we had at least several years left to deepen the work and take everything to the next stage, and to drink many glasses of the wine you so loved along the way.

You were ninety and a force of evolutionary nature.

We communicated several times a day on evolutionary thought or vision. Each letter was clear, potent and reaching for the future. You lived in the future. In so many ways you were a memory of the future human. And in so many ways you were simply human.

Oh my God, I/We will miss you.

Barbara, we will hold a first memorial service for you this Saturday morning at Evolutionary Church. We will send everyone a link tomorrow. But I know you loved a big party.

So, for your central memorial service – we will do exactly what you asked us to do. We will – all of us together throw a big Evolutionary Party, live-streamed online and in person.

We created, together, the Wheel of Co-Creation 2.0. Together we placed "heart's desire"; at the Center of the Wheel of Co-Creation.

Let's Talk About The C Word

At the Evolutionary Party, everyone in your honor, inspired by your calling forth, will speak their heart's desire for the sake of the evolution of love.

Barbara - We promised you we would throw the party - you promised to come.

So, we are counting on you to show up. Tears streaming down my face.

A Great Leader has passed.

A Great Feminine Co-Creator – reborn again and again through what she called Regenopause – a woman who was getting newer every day and never got older – has left our world.

A Great evolutionary has passed.

A great light has gone out in the manifest universe.

But I/We promise you, Barbara, all of us – I/we will continue our EVOLUTIONARY PARTNERSHIP. *Deeper than ever, with more evolutionary joy, with radical commitment, with mad love and delight.*

A great sun has set.

A new sun must now rise.

The torch has been passed. We must all pick it up and light the world on fire.

Evolution must become a revolution. The New story – "evolving the very source code of evolution" is not only possible but urgently necessary as we stand between dystopia and utopia.

Barbara love, do you like what we wrote here, do you want to edit it or rewrite it as you often did with me?

I love you, Barbara. We all love you.

Tender, Audacious, Wondrous, MADLY. Maddening...

You are a blessing.

You are the goodness of evolution pouring into reality. You spoke the word. You were the Logos.

We will continue to speak the word, to tell the story until the world is transformed and every unique self knows they are personal expressions of the evolutionary impulse itself, worthy of infinite dignity, and joy.

All people are born creative. Let us create together - with you guiding us Barbara – from the new world which you are already lighting up.

Tears... Marc Gafni

Books:
52 Code for Conscious Evolution by Barbara Marx Hubbard:
https://amzn.to/33ROAo2

The Biology of Belief by Bruce Lipton:
https://amzn.to/33UmQPB

Science and the Akashic Field: An Integral Theory of Everything by Ervin Laszlo:
https://amzn.to/2KYFSfe

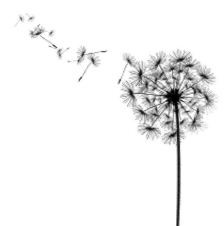

12. Renovating Negativity

When Fatalistic Thoughts Take Hold

The concept that negative thinking is unhealthy isn't groundbreaking. Most of us, at one time or another, have fallen prey to pessimistic thinking, sinking us into a pit of damaging thoughts. The amount of time we sit in that hole is in part due to our belief system of how to handle negativity, our coping habits learned through the family, community, social structures and the strategies we mirror consciously or subconsciously through those around us.

We also have DNA to thank for a portion of our pessimistic or fearful thinking. It's actually inherent to the human animal. Negative thinking tends to be a default response when we are in stressful or dangerous situations. Illness is definitely a circumstance involving stress and fear. We have not evolved far from the prehistoric model of negative thinking. This type of thinking kept our ancestors safe from harm, due to the fact they were constantly in fear of being eaten by the animals around them.

We no longer have the same dangers, yet because our minds

have not evolved, we continue to be triggered by fear and stresses, our bodies naturally revert to the worst-case scenario. Of course, we have evolved in countless other ways, and we have the option to accept or reject these prehistoric behaviours.

The trick is releasing yourself from these primordial, *unconscious reactions*, is becoming aware of how we as individuals respond when our mind perceives physical or emotional danger. This awareness demonstrates to us how to take appropriate and decisive action to alter them. Often our responses are so deeply rooted in our belief system, we fail to notice they are running our lives.

There are a few ways to detect our unconscious habits to stress.

Take an inventory of how you typically respond to negative situations. This will give you a reasonably accurate estimate as to how you are *pre-programmed* when it comes to stressful events. When you have similar reactions to negative events, repeatedly, without awareness, you can be fairly certain this is an underlying response. It might be necessary to ask someone you trust how you consistently respond when you are in stress. Often, we are unaware of our unconscious reactions. Don't be surprised if they tell you things you do not want to hear.

Keep in mind these reactions are based in part on a programmed believe system, habitual reactions as well as conditioned responses. They have either worked or failed us in the past, the funny thing is, even when we have a behaviour that is not working for us, until we reprogram it, when stress, fear, embarrassment, low self-esteem or any number of similar reactions that confront us, we react habitually. Of course, nothing is one hundred percent negative or positive, there are times when these pre-programmed reactions are exactly what we want. We need to decipher if our unconscious reactions serve us. I don't know about you, but I'm not comfortable knowing I'm at the mercy of pre-programmed responses, that I didn't choose, either from genetics, family, society, or my history. I'd like to have more control over this area of my life. I can think of several times when I've reacted unconsciously, and those reactions have caused me embarrassment, shame, and the loss of respect and/or friendships.

The good news, by becoming aware of negative or fatalistic thinking is step one toward changing it. Since awareness is a vital key you will need to pay attention to your actions/reactions. This step is tricky because, at times, we humans are unaware of how we react, or we are too busy blaming others for negative or uncomfortable events in our lives.

Take a moment to consider if you are reacting with cognitive distortions:

Cognitive distortions are simply the ways in which our mind convinces us of something that isn't really true. These inaccurate thoughts are usually used to reinforce negative thinking or emotions telling us things that sound rational and accurate, but really, they only serve to keep us feeling bad about ourselves or our current situation.

By learning to correctly identify this kind of negative thought process, you are able to answer the negative thinking and in turn, invalidate it. By refuting the negative thinking over and over again, it will diminish and be automatically replaced with rational, balanced thinking. It's an ongoing process, keep in mind you are dealing with long-established habits that mostly feel comfortable. They are effortless and therefore easy to allow. With time, practice, and close attention, you will replace the old habits with new ones that serve you. You train yourself to be in control, not the habitual *cognitive distortions* controlling you.

Aaron T Beck first proposed the theory behind *cognitive distortions* in the early 1960s and David D Burns was responsible for popularizing it with common names and examples for the distortions in his 1989 book:

Filtering

We take the negative details and magnify them while filtering out (the) positive aspects of a situation. For instance, a person may pick out a single, unpleasant detail and dwell on it exclusively so that their vision of reality becomes darkened or distorted.

Polarized Thinking or "Black and White" Thinking

In polarized thinking, things are either "black-or-white." We have to be perfect or we're a failure – there is no middle ground. You place people or situations in "either/or" categories, with no shades of gray or allowing for the complexity of most people and situations. If your performance falls short of perfect, you see yourself as a total failure.

Overgeneralization

In this cognitive distortion, we come to a general conclusion based on a single incident or a single piece of evidence. If something bad happens only once, we expect it to happen over and over again. A person may see a single, unpleasant event as part of a never-ending pattern of defeat.

Jumping to Conclusions

Without individuals saying so, we know what they are feeling and why they act the way they do. In particular, we are able to

186

determine how people are feeling toward us.

For example, a person may conclude that someone is reacting negatively toward them but doesn't actually bother to find out if they are correct. Another example is a person may anticipate that things will turn out badly and will feel convinced that their prediction is already an established fact.

Catastrophizing

We expect disaster to strike, no matter what. This is also referred to as "magnifying or minimizing." We hear about a problem and use *what-if* questions (e.g., "What if tragedy strikes?" "What if it happens to me?").

For example, a person might exaggerate the importance of insignificant events (such as their mistake, or someone else's achievement that spikes jealousy within). Or they may inappropriately shrink the magnitude of significant events until they appear tiny (for example, a person's own desirable qualities or someone else's perceived imperfections).

Personalization

Personalization is a distortion in which a person believes that everything others do or say is some kind of direct, personal reaction to the individual person. We also compare ourselves to others trying to determine who is healthier, fitter, et cetera.

Control Fallacies:
Externally Control vs Internal Control

If we feel *externally controlled*, we see ourselves as a helpless victim of fate. For example, "I can't help it if the quality of the work is poor, my boss demanded I work overtime on it."

The fallacy of internal control has us assuming responsibility for the pain and happiness of everyone around us. For example, "Why aren't you happy? Is it because of something I did?"

The Fallacy of Fairness

We feel resentful because we think we know what is fair, but other people won't agree with us. As our parents tell us when we're growing up and something doesn't go our way, "Life isn't always fair." People who go through life applying a measuring ruler against every situation judging its "fairness" will often feel badly and negative because of it. Because life isn't "fair" – things will not always work out in your favour, even when you think they should.

Blaming

We hold other people responsible for our pain or take the other track and blame ourselves for every problem. For example, "Stop making me feel bad about myself!" Nobody can "make" us feel any particular way – only we have control over our own emotions and emotional reactions.

Should-ing On Yourself

We have a list of ironclad rules about how others and ourselves should behave. People who break the rules make us angry, and we feel guilty when we violate these rules. A person may often believe they are trying to motivate themselves with should-have and should-not, as if they have to be punished before they can do anything.

For example, "I really should exercise. I shouldn't be so lazy." *Musts and oughts* are also offenders. The emotional consequence is guilt. When a person directs *should statement's* toward others, they often feel anger, frustration, and resentment.

Emotional Reasoning

We believe that what we feel must be true automatically. If we feel stupid and boring, then we must be stupid and boring. You assume that your unhealthy emotions reflect the way things really are – "I feel it, therefore it must be true."

The Fallacy of Change

We expect that other people will change to suit us if we just pressure or cajole them enough. We need to change people because our hopes for happiness seem to depend entirely on them.

Global Labeling

We generalize one or two qualities into a negative global judgment. These are extreme forms of generalizing and are also referred to as "labeling" and "mislabeling." Instead of describing an error in the context of a specific situation, a person will attach an unhealthy label to themselves.

For example, they may say, "I'm a loser" in a situation where they failed at a specific task. When someone else's behaviour rubs a person the wrong way, they may attach an unhealthy label to him, such as "He's a real jerk." Mislabeling involves describing an event with language that is highly coloured and emotionally loaded. For example, instead of saying someone drops their children off at daycare every day, a person who is mislabeling might say that "they abandon their children to strangers."

Always Being Right

We are continually on trial to prove that our opinions and actions are correct. Being wrong is unthinkable and we will go to any length to demonstrate our rightness. For example, "I don't care how badly arguing with me makes you feel, I'm going to win this argument no matter what because I'm right." Being right of one out of ten times is more important than the feelings of others around a person who engages in this cognitive distortion, even loved ones.

Heaven's Reward Fallacy

We expect our sacrifice and self-denial to pay off as if someone is keeping score. We feel bitter when the reward doesn't come.

Fixing Cognitive Distortions

Cognitive distortions have a way of playing havoc with our lives. If we let them. This kind of *stinkin' thinkin'* can be *undone*, but it takes effort and practice — every day. If you want to stop the irrational thinking, you can start by implementing the exercises below.

Identify Our Cognitive Distortion

We need to create a list of our troublesome thoughts and examine them later for matches with a list of cognitive distortions. An examination of our cognitive distortions allows us to see which distortions we prefer. Additionally, this process will allow us to think about our problem or predicament in more natural and realistic ways.

Examine the Evidence

A thorough examination of experience allows us to identify the basis for our distorted thoughts. If we are quite self-critical, then, we should identify a number of experiences and situations where we had success.

Double Standard Method

An alternative to "self-talk" that is harsh, and demeaning is to talk to ourselves in the same compassionate and caring way that we would talk with a friend in a similar situation.

Thinking in Shades of Gray

Instead of thinking about our problem or predicament in an either/or polarity, evaluate things on a scale of 0-100. When a plan or goal is not fully realized, think about and evaluate the experience as a partial success, again, on a scale of 0-100.

Survey Method

We need to seek the opinions of others regarding whether our thoughts and attitudes are realistic. If we believe that our anxiety about an upcoming event is unwarranted, check with a few trusted friends or relatives.

Definitions

What does it mean to define ourselves as "inferior," "a loser," "a fool," or "abnormal." An examination of these and other global labels likely will reveal that they more closely represent specific behaviours, or an identifiable behaviour pattern instead of the total person. This begs the question, "What is normal?"

Re-attribution

Often, we automatically blame ourselves for the problems and predicaments we experience. Identify external factors and other individuals that contributed to the problem. Regardless of the degree of responsibility we assume, our energy is best utilized in the pursuit of resolutions to problems or identifying ways to cope with predicaments.

Cost-Benefit Analysis

It is helpful to list the advantages and disadvantages of feelings, thoughts, or behaviours. A cost-benefit analysis will help us to ascertain what we are gaining from feeling badly, from distorted thinking, and from inappropriate behaviour.

If you recognize yourself in any of these descriptions and want to delve deeper into cognitive distortions and how to overcome them, I recommend you read David D. Burns book: *Feeling Good: The New Mood Therapy.*

Reference:

David D Burns, D.D. (1989) New York: William Morrow
The feeling good handbook: Using the new mood therapy in everyday life
https://amzn.to/31X8L28

Fixing Cognitive Distortions References:
Beck, A. T. (1976) Cognitive therapies and emotional disorders. New York: New American Library Burns, D. D. (1980)

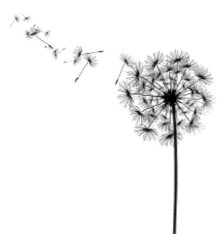

13. Protection from Within

The Delete Button

Your mind, like a computer, it has an InBox, a place for JunkMail, and a Delete Button. Not all the information accessible to you from outside sources is valid or appreciated. After a cancer diagnosis, it will be imperative for you to continuously filter the in-formation coming into your *well-being* file.

You will be inundated with advice offered by well-meaning friends, family, relatives and just about anyone with access to you, either in person or via social media. You'll receive positive AND negative scenarios, designed to educate you during this firestorm of medical statistics, conflicting data, ambiguous percentages and frightening probabilities.

Guidance will come to you from expected as well as unexpected sources. As if having cancer weren't enough, it will be necessary for you to navigate a minefield of opinions administered by those with and without direct cancer experience. I urge you to read with caution, listen to your own intuition when it comes to what others are advising.

Never forget this is YOUR illness and you have rights. Unfortunately, you will be required to take aggressive action when it comes to unsolicited recommendations in regard to your treatment choices. Don't be surprised to find yourself singled out and made responsible for both getting sick and the choices you make regarding treatment and recovery.

Others think they are helping when in fact they are adding to your stress at a time when undue pressure causes your immune system to slow down. Their well-meaning stories and counsel can in fact move you into a place of fear, inertia, and depression.

No two cancers are alike, and every person responds in accordance with variables too numerous to list. Torturing yourself by listening to information not pertaining to you will not serve you in the long run. Filtering out unwanted data does not constitute reckless negligent behaviour on your part, it is simply a coping strategy against unwanted trash cluttering the inbox of your healing.

The healthy course of action will be to listen to your inner voice. What is it telling you about how you are feeling emotionally, and are you able to appropriately process information in this moment? Your ability to filter information will change from day to day and often moment to moment. This is not about ignoring the facts, it is a strategy to keep you sane and ultimately healthy.

Surrounding yourself with a trusted team of loved ones who can advocate on your behalf, will serve you in the long run. One or two people, at most, who keep track of your appointments, your test results and your chosen course of action. This is not always available to everyone, but if possible, search out an advocate who will speak and filter on your behalf.

Joanna Montogomery, a cancer thriver and writer gives examples of her experiences after her diagnosis:

"I've been dealing with metastatic cancer for going on 5 years now, and I've tried a lot of remedies, from the traditional to the holistic and everything in between. But I haven't, nor will I ever, put all my eggs in one basket. Why does it have to be either/or?

Must the practices of eating a clean diet of whole foods and taking medically proven cancer treatments to be mutually exclusive? And who am I to call myself an expert and tell others, particularly those in life or death situations, what to do?"

Joanna continues: "When I was first diagnosed, I was bombarded with fervent endorsements for various cancer remedies, and the claims sounded wonderfully promising."

"Cancer can't live in an alkaline environment...if you drink alkaline water and eat foods that have low acid Ph, cancer won't be able to live in your body."

"Cannabis oil is a cure for cancer." "Turmeric/curcumin kills cancer cells."

"Frankincense is more effective than chemotherapy at treating some cancers."

"Cutting all sugar out of your diet will cause your cancer to die."

"Have the courage to REFUSE chemo and you will have a better chance of living to 100."

"It is NOT a cancer 'battle' when you put all four paws in the air and blindly and stupidly trust the cancer industry."

"Chemo is an over-priced highly ineffective chemical attack on your immune system which if it was healthy, to BEGIN with, you would have never gotten cancer at all."

"When you're ready to stop poisoning yourself, the real, natural cure is out there."

"If you were evolved enough to recognize the truth about the pharmaceutical industry, you wouldn't be risking leaving your daughter without a mother."

"You are part of the problem, a pawn for the cancer machine."

The list of purported "cures" out there is long and growing. And, of course, a cancer diagnosis is the quickest way to get a desperate patient (or their loved ones) to start seeking magic solutions and cure-alls. We'll try most anything, and possibly even spend our last hours and dollars doing so.

The phrase "if it sounds too good to be true, it probably is" comes to mind right now.

For me personally, I have chosen to cover as many bases as I can. I've tried several different types of chemotherapy drugs. I've participated in a clinical trial. I've had surgeries. I've done infusions as well as oral treatments. I've given myself injections. I've changed my diet. I buy whole, organic foods. I avoid processed foods and toxic chemicals. I drink green tea instead of coffee (usually). I watch my sugar intake. Our family drinks only alkaline water. I soak in Himalayan sea salt. I consume a variety of supplements and oils.

There's an overwhelming amount of information out there. And those of us battling potentially terminal illnesses would love nothing more than for a miracle cure to be found.

In fact, some of us are so desperate that we'll spend our last dollars and our last days chasing that so-called miracle.

I'm not immune to it either. Although I chose traditional medicine to fight my cancer, surgery followed by 24 rounds of aggressive chemotherapy, I have supplemented it with tons of holistic remedies and treatments. My view has been that if it can't hurt me and has been reported to shrink tumors and make cancer disappear, what do I have to lose?

Toni Bernhard J.D from *Psychology Today* who wrote:
4 Tips for Dealing with Unsolicited Health Advice gives these recommendations:

Shove it under the bed (literally or metaphorically)

Twenty years ago, my dear friend Anne was in the final stages of cancer. She was a therapist by profession, but she decided to see one herself to help her cope with what was happening.

One of her ongoing difficulties was that almost everyone who came to visit brought her some kind of treatment, whether it be a supplement, an herbal tea, or a crystal to wear around her neck. She told me that sometimes she wanted to scream: "I'm in the hands of good doctors; we're doing everything we can to keep me alive; I don't want or need your advice!" But she didn't because she didn't want to hurt people who were being kind enough to visit.

When Anne raised this dilemma at a counseling session, her therapist suggested that she smile and say, "Thank you very much," and put the item down. Then, as soon as the visit was over and the person had left, shove it under your bed. It turned out to be just the advice she needed.

I've found this to be a valuable strategy. When I get unsolicited advice via email or a private Facebook message, sometimes I answer by simply saying, "Thanks for thinking of me." And that's it; I purposefully don't address the substance of the advice. I've found that if I engage someone on a suggestion that's clearly off-base for me by responding with something like, "Thanks, but I'm aware of that treatment and I'm sure it won't work for me," it invites the person to continue the dialogue – sometimes to try even harder to convince me that he or she is right. I don't want to have to defend my treatment decisions; it takes up too much of what precious little energy I have. So, as an act of self-protection and self-compassion, I answer politely, but briefly, and avoid addressing what the person is suggesting that I do. In other words, I metaphorically shove it under the bed.

Ignore it

This strategy is often only available when, unlike in the example above with Anne, the unsolicited advice arrives in a non-person-to- person interaction – via an email or in a Facebook comment for example. In those circumstances, you can always choose not to respond at all.

I used to answer every single online communication that came my way (and I still do if it's about my books or other writing). Now, if it's unsolicited health advice, even though I appreciate that people are trying to help, I admit that I might simply ignore it.

For example, one person told me to forgo all future breast cancer treatments and start eating lemons because acid kills cancer. That's a piece of unsolicited advice I decided not to respond to. If that person is reading this, please understand that I appreciate that you were thinking of me, but I consulted multiple doctors and spent many hours online doing research before I settled on a treatment plan. It's better for my peace of mind not to second guess that plan unless some change in my health requires reevaluating it.

Be honest about how you feel about being given unsolicited advice

This is an especially good option to consider when you're offered in-person advice from well-meaning family and friends. I've been given lots of health advice that's of no use to me whatsoever. I often just mumble, "Thanks," but sometimes I muster the courage to say: "I appreciate your attempt to help, but I'd rather talk about something other than my health"; or "I appreciate your suggestion, but my doctor and I already have a treatment plan and I want to stick to it."

To my surprise, so far, this response has been well-received. I think I know why. Family and friends who offer unsolicited advice have the best of intentions. Their hearts are in the right place: they're as frustrated as I am that I'm chronically ill. And so, when I get up the nerve to be honest with them about not wanting unsolicited advice, they're actually relieved, as if they'd felt obligated to try and help in this way but have been let off the hook.

Being honest may not always be the best strategy, but I'd keep it in mind as a possibility. Let's face it, some family and friends can't resist giving advice or bringing us cures. For them, that "Thank you" followed by shoving it under the bed (metaphorically or literally) works better.

Work on accepting that people won't always behave the way you want them to.

This is good advice for everyone, whether chronically ill or not. We can't control other people's behavior. Despite our attempts to be honest with family and friends about not wanting advice, as I mentioned above, some may continue to give it. This calls for self-protection in the form of compassion for ourselves. We can gently remind ourselves what a burden it is to have to add to our ongoing pain and illness the work of having to access how to skillfully deal with what others are telling us to do about our health.

Dealing with unsolicited advice also calls for equanimity. This means, first, accepting that people won't always treat us the way we want them to and, second, having that be okay with us. This is the essence of equanimity – being okay with our life as it is, knowing it won't always be pleasant and it won't always unfold the way we'd like it to.

Cancer care is a highly volatile and confusing time that is inundated with the latest therapies, holistic approaches, dietary options, western vs homeopathic medicine, to name just a few. The last thing you or your family needs at this time, is a curious neighbour or co-worker, recounting horror stories of their cousin's best friend's fathers experience with cancer. You've earned the right to say, "no more!" The right to say, "I refuse to listen, and I want you to stop talking...immediately!"

This is a time to be fierce with unsolicited information. If you are unable to quell the advice in person, try explaining you are having an extremely difficult day and are overwhelmed at the moment. Instruct them to write out their findings in an email and you will read it when you have the mental and physical energy. When the email arrives: You have options:

- ✓ Read it or save it for a time when you are better equipped to filter.
- ✓ Send it to a friend, family member, or advocate, who can decipher it for you; and, if necessary, move it to the trash folder.
- ✓ Most importantly, move on with no regrets.

I personally love the instinctive advice from Susan Silk and Barry Goldman, in their book called *The Ring Theory*. It is a brilliant piece of advice for everyone who has someone in their life with an illness, the loss of a loved one, or stress of any kind.

The Ring Theory – How to Not Say the Wrong Thing
by Susan Silk and Barry Goldman April 07, 2013 Los Angeles Times

When Susan had breast cancer, we heard a lot of lame remarks, but our favourite came from one of Susan's colleagues. She wanted, she needed, to visit Susan after the surgery, but Susan didn't feel like having visitors, and she said so. Her colleague's response? "This isn't just about you."

"It's not?" Susan wondered. "My breast cancer is not about me? It's about you?"

The same theme came up again when our friend Katie had a brain aneurysm. She was in intensive care for a long time and finally got out and into a step-down unit. She was no longer covered with tubes and lines and monitors, but she was still in rough shape. A friend came and saw her and then stepped into the hall with Katie's husband, Pat. "I wasn't prepared for this," she told him. "I don't know if I can handle it."

This woman loves Katie, and she said what she did because the sight of Katie in this condition moved her so deeply. But it was the wrong thing to say. And it was wrong in the same way Susan's colleague's remark was wrong.

Susan has since developed a simple technique to help people avoid this mistake. It works for all kinds of crises: medical, legal, financial, romantic, even existential. She calls it the Ring Theory.

Draw a circle. This is the centre ring. In it, put the name of the person at the centre of the current trauma. For Katie's aneurysm, that's Katie.

Now draw a larger circle around the first one. In that ring put the name of the person next closest to the trauma. In the case of Katie's aneurysm, that was Katie's husband, Pat.

Repeat the process as many times as you need to. In each larger ring put the next closest people. Parents and children before more distant relatives. Intimate friends in smaller rings, less intimate friends in larger ones. When you are done, you have what is referred to as a "kvetching order". One of Susan's patients found it useful to tape it to her refrigerator.

Here are the rules:
The person in the centre ring can say anything she wants to anyone, anywhere. She can kvetch (Yiddish word for chronic complaining) and complain and whine and moan and curse the heavens and say, "Life is unfair" and "Why me?" That's the one payoff for being in the centre ring.

Everyone else can say those things too, but only to people in larger rings.

When you are talking to a person in a ring smaller than yours, someone closer to the centre of the crisis, the goal is to help. Listening is often more helpful than talking. But if you're going to open your mouth, ask yourself if what you are about to say is likely to provide comfort and support. If it isn't, don't say it. Don't, for example, give advice. People who are suffering from trauma don't need advice. They need comfort and support. So say, "I'm sorry" or "This must be really hard on you" or "Can I bring you a pot roast?" Don't say, "You should hear what happened to me" or "Here's what I would do if I were you." And don't (ever) say, "This is really bringing me down."

If you want to scream or cry or complain, if you want to tell someone how shocked you are or how icky you feel, or whine about how it reminds you of all the terrible things that have happened to you lately, that's fine. It's a perfectly normal response. Just do it to someone in a bigger ring.

Comfort – IN, dump OUT.

There was nothing wrong with Katie's friend saying she was not prepared for how horrible Katie looked, or even that she didn't think she could handle it. The mistake was that she said those things to Pat. She dumped IN.

Complaining to someone in a smaller ring than yours doesn't do either of you any good. On the other hand, being supportive of her principal caregiver may be the best thing you can do for the patient.

Most of us know this. Almost nobody would complain to the patient about how rotten she looks. Almost no one would say that looking at her makes them think of the fragility of life and their own closeness to death. In other words, we know enough not to dump into the centre ring. The Ring Theory merely expands that intuition and makes it more concrete: Don't just avoid dumping into the centre ring, avoid dumping into any ring smaller than your own.

Remember, you can say whatever you want if you just wait until you're talking to someone in a larger ring than yours.

It works in all kinds of crises – medical, legal, even existential. It's the 'Ring Theory' of kvetching. The first rule is comfort in, dump out.

Susan Silk is a clinical psychologist. Barry Goldman is an arbitrator and mediator and the author of *"The Science of Settlement: Ideas for Negotiators."*

The Ring Theory - Susan Silk-Los Angeles Times:
https://www.latimes.com/nation/la-oe-0407-silk-ring-theory-20130407-story.html

How to Deal with Unsolicited Advice - Tony Bernhard J.D.:
https://www.psychologytoday.com/ca/blog/turning-straw-gold/201507/4-tips-dealing-unsolicited-health-advice

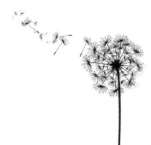

14. How Gratitude Changes People

An Informative Approach

I've been studying and writing on the positive energy of gratitude for the past five years. It's a passion project that touches all areas of my life. I write a weekly Facebook post on how to cultivate gratitude in your life.

When I walked the Camino de Santiago, from France to Santiago, Spain, I had the words: "What Are You Grateful For" inscribed on my backpack. It opened up interactions and discussions on the value and wisdom of gratitude. Those five words turned my Camino into a true pilgrimage of the soul.

Over the years, I have sought out experts that I go to for science, social and heart-based truth, from various fields who understand how gratitude changes lives. I love science almost as much as the rhythm of our souls. Sadly, gratitude has become a buzzword. Please don't let its popularity dissuade you from the importance of practicing gratitude and allowing it to transform into an exceptional and remarkably simple asset for living a phenomenal life.

I find it fascinating that of all the spiritual masters that I've read or studied over the years an array of suggestions and opinions on how to live a well-rounded life. They disagree on many points and procedures, but they do unanimously agree on one thing...PRACTICING GRATITUDE.

My Favourite go-to science-based expert on gratitude is Robert Emmons, Ph.D. He's a Professor of Psychology at the University of California Davis. Dr. Emmons has been researching and writing on gratitude from the early days. I trust his research. When I'm personally in a place of confusion, the need for hard science becomes vital. My spirituality is such that I don't necessarily question my beliefs, but I do like having science back me up. Below is an essay that Robert Emmons wrote for the online magazine of the *Greater Good Science* Ct. UC Berkeley. It gave me the hard science behind why I need to continue practicing and growing in this area of my life.

Why Gratitude Is Good by Robert Emmons

Gratitude journals and other gratitude practices often seem so simple and basic; in our studies, my colleagues and I often have people keep gratitude journals for just three weeks. And yet the results have been overwhelming. We've studied more than one thousand people, from ages eight to 80, and found that people who practice gratitude consistently report a host of benefits:

Psychological
- ✓ Higher levels of positive emotions
- ✓ More alert, alive, and awake
- ✓ More joy and pleasure
- ✓ More optimism and happiness

Physical

- ✓ Stronger immune systems
- ✓ Less bothered by aches and pains
- ✓ Lower blood pressure
- ✓ Exercise more and take better care of their health
- ✓ Sleep longer and feel more refreshed upon waking

Social

- ✓ More helpful, generous, and compassionate
- ✓ More forgiving
- ✓ More outgoing
- ✓ Feel less lonely and isolated

So, what's really behind our research results – why might gratitude have these transformative effects on people's lives?

I think there are several important reasons, but I want to highlight four in particular.

1. *Gratitude allows us to celebrate the present.*
It magnifies positive emotions.

Gratitude Image Research on emotion shows that positive emotions wear off quickly. Our emotional systems like newness. They like novelty. They like change. We adapt to positive life circumstances so that before too long, the new car, the new spouse, the new house – they don't feel so new and exciting anymore.

But gratitude makes us appreciate the value of something, and when we appreciate the value of something, we extract more benefits from it; we're less likely to take it for granted.

In effect, I think gratitude allows us to participate more in life. We notice the positives more, and that magnifies the pleasure you get from life. Instead of adapting to goodness, we celebrate goodness. We spend so much time watching things—movies, computer screens, sports—but with gratitude, we become greater participants in our lives as opposed to spectators.

2. Gratitude blocks toxic, negative emotions, such as envy, resentment, regret.

Emotions that can destroy our happiness. There's even recent evidence, including a 2008 study by psychologist Alex Wood in the Journal of Research in Personality, showing that gratitude can reduce the frequency and duration of episodes of depression.

***This makes sense:** You cannot feel envious and grateful at the same time. They're incompatible feelings. If you're grateful, you can't resent someone for having something that you don't. Those are very different ways of relating to the world, and sure enough, the research I've done with colleagues Michael McCullough and JoAnn Tsang have suggested that people who have high levels of gratitude have low levels of resentment and envy.*

3. Grateful people are more stress resistant.

There's a number of studies showing that in the face of serious trauma, adversity, and suffering if people have a grateful disposition, they'll recover more quickly. I believe gratitude gives people a perspective from which they can interpret negative life events and help them guard against post-traumatic stress and lasting anxiety.

4. Grateful people have a higher sense of self-worth.

I think that's because when you're grateful, you have the sense that someone else is looking out for you – someone else has provided for your well-being, or you notice a network of relationships, past and present, of people who are responsible for helping you get to where you are right now.

Once you start to recognize the contributions that other people have made to your life – once you realize that other people have seen the value in you – you can transform the way you see yourself.

Challenges to gratitude

Just because gratitude is good doesn't mean it's always easy. Practicing gratitude can be at odds with some deeply ingrained psychological tendencies.

Give Thanks image One is the "self-serving bias." That means that when good things happen to us, we attribute them to something we did, but when bad things happen, we blame other people or circumstances.

Gratitude really goes against the self-serving bias because when we're grateful, we give credit to other people for our success. We accomplished some of it ourselves, yes, but we widen our range of attribution to also say, "Well, my parents gave me this opportunity." Or, "I had teachers. I had mentors. I had siblings, peers – other people assisted me along the way." That's very different from a self-serving bias.

Gratitude also goes against our need to feel in control of our environment. Sometimes with gratitude, you just have to accept life as it is and be grateful for what you have.

Finally, gratitude contradicts the "just-world" hypothesis, which says that we get what we deserve in life. Good things happen to good people, bad things happen to bad people. But it doesn't always work out that way, does it? Bad things happen to good people and vice versa.

With gratitude comes the realization that we get more than we deserve. I'll never forget the comment by a man at a talk I gave on gratitude. "It's a good thing we don't get what we deserve," he said. "I'm grateful because I get far more than I deserve."

This goes against a message we get a lot in our contemporary culture: that we deserve the good fortune that comes our way, that we're entitled to it. If you deserve everything, if you're entitled to everything, it makes it a lot harder to be grateful for anything.

How to Cultivate Gratitude

Partly because these challenges to gratitude can be so difficult to overcome, I get asked a lot about how we can go beyond just occasionally feeling more grateful to actually becoming a more grateful person.

I detail many steps for cultivating gratitude in my book, Thanks! and summarize many of them in this Greater Good article. I should add, though, that despite the fact that I've been studying gratitude for 11 years and know all about it, I still find that I have to put a lot of conscious effort into practicing gratitude. In fact, my wife says, "How is it that you're supposed to be this huge expert on gratitude? You're the least grateful person I know!" Well, she has a point because it's easy to lapse into a negativity mindset. But these are some of the specific steps I like to recommend for overcoming the challenges to gratitude.

First is to keep a gratitude journal, as I've had people do in my experiments. This can mean listing just five things for which you're grateful every week. This practice works, I think, because it consciously, intentionally focuses our attention on developing more grateful thinking and on eliminating ungrateful thoughts. It helps guard against taking things for granted; instead, we see gifts in life as new and exciting. I do believe that people who live a life of pervasive thankfulness really do experience life differently than people who cheat themselves out of life by not feeling grateful.

Similarly, another gratitude exercise is to practice counting your blessings *on a regular basis, maybe first thing in the morning, maybe in the evening. What are you grateful for today? You don't have to write them down on paper. (although writing them down is an effective practice to strengthen your gratitude and shift healing to the next level)*

You can also use concrete reminders to practice gratitude, *which can be particularly effective in working with children, who aren't abstract thinkers like adults are. For instance, I read about a woman in Vancouver whose family developed this practice of putting money in "gratitude jars." At the end of the day, they emptied their pockets and put spare change in those jars. They had a regular reminder, a routine, to get them to focus on gratitude. Then, when the jar became full, they gave the money in it to a needy person or a good cause within their community.*

Practices like this can not only teach children the importance of gratitude but can show that gratitude impels people to "pay it for-ward"– to give to others in some measure as they themselves have received.

Finally, I think it's important to think outside of the box when *it comes to gratitude. Mother Theresa talked about how grateful she was to the people she was helping, the sick and dying in the slums of Calcutta because they enabled her to grow and deepen her spirituality. That's a very different way of thinking about gratitude – gratitude for what we can give as opposed to what we receive. But that can be a very powerful way of cultivating a sense of gratitude.*

Thanks! How Practicing Gratitude Can Make You Happier
Dr. Emmons: <u>https://amzn.to/31U16UQ</u>

Why I Practice Gratitude

By cultivating and writing about gratitude, my life has improved because of it, and when you see improvement, why not ramp it up a level?

In addition to the above suggestions by Dr. Emmons, I've added the step of offering gratitude to complete strangers. It could be as simple as telling a barista that the latte he prepared for me made my day brighter. Or complementing the Fedex driver on his professionalism. Anything is fair game.

An additional bonus to cultivating an attitude of gratitude is when I catch myself about to get impatient with someone, I calm my reaction and imagine what it would be like to be in their shoes. Gratitude helps me consider how I'd want to be treated if the roles were reversed. It's easier to achieve this from a place of calm, to act instead of *react*. Do I always succeed? Absolutely not, but I have discovered that through practicing and from years of searching for opportunities to be grateful, I've gained and understanding and ability to calm judgements, anger, or negative thoughts. I'm more in control of my emotions and have more joy in my life through the simple act of gratitude.

Gratitude has far-reaching effects. Keep trying, growing, and evolving with it. Your life, your health, the lives of those around you, and your day to day living will be a miracle in its sweetness.

On that note, it is with deep gratitude I send this book, my "baby", out into the world. My wish is that it lands in the hands of those who need it.

It was a delight to interview the people in this book, they not only have inspired me, they changed the way I live my life. I feel honoured and privileged to have met them. They put their trust in me and for that I will be forever grateful.

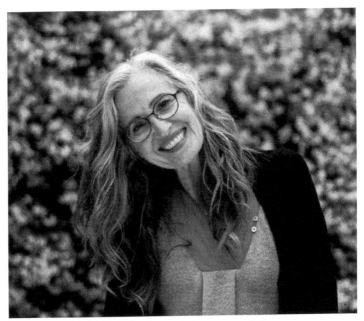

Shauna Marie MacDonald

Shauna Marie's inherent need for expression emerged by way of the custom home building company she operated with her husband Ron for 26 years. Designing and decorating homes became her creative outlet while raising three daughters.

After Shauna Marie's divorce and their children had grown, the evolution of new and exciting outlets of expression emerged: Travel, Interaction and Writing.

In 2011 Shauna Marie explored Europe for ten months. This pivotal experience opened new doors of creativity by way of the written word and communicating with people from diverse cultures and backgrounds.

Shauna Marie MacDonald

A native Canadian, Shauna Marie currently resides in Calgary, Canada near her eldest daughter, cherished grandchildren and friends. Yearly trips to visit her other daughters and grandchildren in St. Louis, USA and Barcelona, Spain enable Shauna Marie to connect with family and indulge her passion for travel.

Shauna Marie's writing and coaching pursuits evolved naturally by way of sharing her unique take on living in her beloved Italy. Walking 800 km through France and Spain along the Camino de Santiago Trail. The one million steps along the trail gave her the opportunity to ask what others felt about life all the while listening and being guided by her own inner wisdom.

Let's Talk About The C Word – How Cancer Gave More Than It Took, stems from the loss of Shauna's ex-husband Ron from cancer. During the final days of his life, he shared a profound realization that for him "Cancer Gave More Than It Took".

Shauna Marie began researching scientifically proven and effective wholistic processes to alleviate the fear associated with cancer, Shauna Marie coaches her clients on ways to bridge the gap between fear and happiness through *The 8 Essential Pillars to a Happy and Healthy Life.*

Facebook: https://www.facebook.com/shaunamarie8
LinkedIn: https://www.linkedin.com/in/shaunamariedesigns/din
Twitter: https://twitter.com/ShaunaMarieMacD
Instagram: https://www.instagram.com/shauna.marie1/

Apply for a 30-minute conversation with Shauna Marie
www.shaunamarie.ca/application

Ultimate Life Mastery – 8 Essential Pillars Course
www.ShaunaMarie.ca

Medical Disclaimer: Always consult your physician before beginning any auxiliary health and wellness program. This general information is not intended to diagnose any medical condition or to replace your healthcare professional. Consult with your healthcare professional to design an appropriate health and wellness prescription. If you experience any pain or difficulty with these practices, stop and consult your healthcare provider.

Made in the USA
Middletown, DE
30 September 2019